Make Your Own

Perfume

Make Your Own

Perfume

SALLY HORNSEY

A HOW TO BOOK

ROBINSON

ROBINSON

First published in the UK in 2011 by Spring Hill, an imprint of How To Books Ltd

Reprinted in 2017 by Robinson

5 7 9 10 8 6

Copyright © Sally Hornsey, 2011

The moral right of the author has been asserted.

A CIP catalogue record for this book
is available from the British Library.

ISBN: 978-1-90586-269-6

Printed and bound in Great Britain by
Clays Ltd, Elcograf S.p.A.

Designed and typeset by Mousemat Design Ltd

Papers used by Robinson are from well-managed forests
and other responsible sources

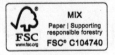

Robinson
An imprint of
Little, Brown Book Group
Carmelite House
50 Victoria Embankment
London EC4Y 0DZ

An Hachette UK Company
www.hachette.co.uk

www.littlebrown.co.uk

How To Books are published by Robinson, an imprint of Little, Brown Book Group. We welcome proposals from authors who have first-hand experience of their subjects. Please set out the aims of your book, its target market and its suggested contents in an email to howtobooks@littlebrown.co.uk

Dedication

This book is dedicated to my late father,
who grew the roses that enabled me to make my first perfume,
and to my wonderful mother, even though she refused to wear it!

Contents

Acknowledgements

My heartfelt thanks go out to everyone who helped me find the time for the big book-writing sessions. To my lovely team at Plush Folly, who held the fort, hardly noticing I was missing! To my family, for patiently becoming self-sufficient when they wanted to eat, and to my very kind husband, for providing me with the aroma of peanut butter on toast.

A special thanks to Nickie at Plush Folly, for her help in hunting out most of the photos; to Tara, for letting me use her wonderful collection of perfume bottles; and to Jo, for filling our office with the most beautiful smells. You're all great!

No elegance is possible without perfume.
It is the unseen, unforgettable,
ultimate accessory.

Coco Chanel

Introduction

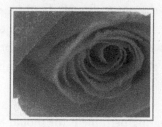

Nearly everything we come into contact with has a smell. From natural aromas such as roast potatoes, a vase of flowers, a tree in blossom, car emissions, roadworks, pencils, paper and skin to synthetic, purpose-made odours such as washing powder, sweets, shampoo, cosmetics, bathroom cleaner and polish ... the list of scents is endless.

Traditionally, a perfumer created a perfume by choosing from a wealth of literally thousands of raw ingredients. A number of these essences were blended together bit by bit, until the desired aroma was achieved. Nowadays, the process is similar, but the ability to isolate components within certain perfume materials, or to create synthetic aromas, enables the perfumer quickly, yet skilfully, to arrive at a desired scent.

Creating a perfume can be an exciting and challenging task – the skills required demand a lot of patience! A critical sense of smell, familiarity with raw materials and their impact on a formulation will come after years of experience and expert guidance, but you can also have an enormous amount of fun and pleasure while you learn.

Olfactory nerves

Practically everything that has an odour will have been considered for inclusion in perfume at one time or other. Good perfumers ferret out anything from the gorgeous to the downright outrageous if it enhances a perfume's overall aroma. From honeydew to whale spew, nothing goes untried.

All aromas have an important role, and these smells are there for a purpose. The olfactory nerves that control our sense of smell register odours and carry them to our brain to trigger certain reactions and feelings. The smell of roast potatoes will make us hungry and produce digestive juices while the synthetic pine scent in bathroom cleaner reminds us of the sensation of the fresh, clean outdoors.

This direct connection with our brains means that our sense of smell is constantly active, even when we are asleep. We cannot choose to ignore a smell in the same way that we can turn a blind eye or a deaf ear to unwanted sights or sounds.

Of all our senses, it is the sense of smell that triggers our strongest memories. For example, catching the scent of a particular perfume may suddenly remind you of a person who often wears it, while the smell of freshly cut grass happily transports me back to my childhood, watching my father mow the lawn.

Choosing a perfume

The ancient custom of wearing perfume is (or should be) a pleasurable experience for everyone. Perfume is a powerful mood-enhancer; it can lift your spirits, evoke pleasant emotions and trigger happy thoughts.

Choosing a different perfume for different occasions should be a personal indulgence enjoyed by all and not limited by the cost of shop-bought designer scents. Making your own perfume and perfumed products is as enjoyable as choosing which perfume to wear. You can design fragrances that are exciting, uplifting, sultry and amorous, or create a variety of perfumes to match your mood, your character and your lifestyle.

Make Your Own Perfume will guide you through a variety of individual aromas, encouraging you to design and assemble your own perfume. It offers a wealth of blending tips and tricks to help you create your own range of gorgeous signature scents and scented products.

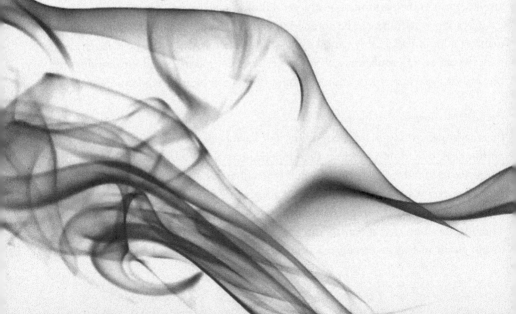

A BRIEF HISTORY OF PERFUME

Perfume and scents have a place in our history, and history books are liberally sprinkled with many references to the use of perfume or scented products. The word 'perfume' is derived from the Latin *per fume*, which means 'through smoke'. This stems from the times when aromatic woods, tree resins and other fragrant bits and pieces were placed on hot coals to enable their wonderful aromas to permeate the air. Today, the word *parfum* appears on cosmetic product labels whenever a fragrance or essential oil blend has been included as part of the ingredients.

Burning incense

One of the oldest uses of perfumed products comes from the burning of incense and tree gum such as frankincense and myrrh used in religious services. The Holy Bible, for example, makes references to gold, frankincense and myrrh being given as expensive and treasured gifts to the infant Jesus by the Three Wise Men.

Ancient Egypt

The Egyptians considered certain aromas to be even more precious than gold, and chose to be buried with specific scents. References to perfume are written in hieroglyphics on ancient Egyptian tombs, where the word for perfume is translated as 'fragrance of the gods'. These early perfumers showed great skill: when a jar of scented balm (unguent) found in a tomb was opened after thousands of years, the aroma from the perfume was still evident and exquisite.

It is no surprise, then, that Cleopatra, Queen of Egypt, was well known for her passion for perfume. When she sailed to greet Mark Antony, it was on a ship carrying perfumed sails – so her arrival was heralded by clouds of perfume even before the vessel came into view!

Ancient Greece

For all the Egyptians' use and love of perfumes, it was the ancient Greeks who made the important link between aromas and their effect on moods and behaviour – the basis of today's practice of aromatherapy. In classical Greece, certain smells were extracted from plants and used as treatments to clear confusion, cure common illnesses and help relieve more unusual disorders. Just as importantly, perfumes were also used as the means to attract love and affection.

Ancient Rome

The Romans, famous for their public baths, also adored the art of wearing perfume, applying scent liberally throughout the day. In fact, it was common practice to cover pet dogs and horses in scent, and caged birds, their wings doused in perfume, were set free to fly through Roman halls in order to allow a fine spray of perfume to fall on the guests below. In Roman society, everything possible was perfumed, including curtains, candles, tablecloths and cushions.

France
In a similar practice, although much later in the sixteenth century, gloves perfumed with herbs, spices and flowers were introduced in France. These enabled men and women to clutch something sweet-smelling to their noses while walking through sewage-ridden city streets. Perfumes were so popular with the French aristocracy that common, everyday items such as wigs, clothing, fans and furniture were doused liberally in scent. It is said that Napoleon used 60 bottles of jasmine oil every month, while Josephine's preferred perfume was musk – so they must have made a very fragrant couple between them!

Germany
One of the first major turning points in perfume history, which took perfume a step forwards from traditional tree resins, herbs, flowers and spices, came about in Cologne, Germany, during the eighteenth century. Johann Maria Farina, a successful perfumer, wanted a lighter, less intense aroma – something more subtle than regular perfumes of the day, yet equally, if not more so, alluring. He blended softer, refreshing oils of bergamot, lemon, neroli (bitter-orange blossom) and rosemary until he had the exact aroma he wanted.

Because the aroma was still too strong, however, he began diluting his blend, first with bathwater, then with wine. While neither practice produced exactly the desired result, this experimentation did lead to success in blending his oils with an alcohol and water base: the first version of *eau de cologne* (literally 'water of Cologne'). This formula is still in use today.

Synthetic ingredients
The biggest development in perfume history has to be the introduction of synthetic ingredients. Traditionally, perfumes were made using natural ingredients extracted from parts of a plant. These, however, were problematic in terms of availability, consistency and reliability; a failed harvest, for instance, could devastate a perfume house.

Towards the end of the nineteenth century, synthetic ingredients were developed. These had no link to natural counterparts such as rose, jasmine and violet, yet they smelled flowery and sweet, just like the real thing. This invention of organic chemistry revolutionised the business of perfumery. Suddenly, synthetic perfume products could be used in place of hard-to-find, difficult-to-cultivate or expensive ingredients, allowing perfume developers much more freedom in the products they could create.

In addition, synthetic compounds provided fragrances not found in nature. For instance, calone, a synthetic compound also known as methylbenzodioxepinone, is a clean, metallic, ozone-fresh, salty/marine scent that is widely used in perfumes today.

It was in 1921 that Coco Chanel launched her own brand of perfume called Chanel No 5. When presented with a number of samples, she reportedly stated that her favourite was 'number 5'– hence the name of the infamous perfume that we know and (some of us) love. Chanel No 5 was created by perfumer Ernest Beaux, who was the first to use synthetic aldehydes (organic alcohol-based compounds) in perfumery. In fact, Chanel No 5 was the first completely synthetic mass-market fragrance.

Before the advent of synthetic components, perfumes were a luxury item: they were expensive and only the rich could easily afford them. As synthetic materials became more easily obtainable and less expensive, fashion designers and cosmetic houses gradually turned their attention to designing perfumes manufactured en masse, thereby making them more affordable – and available – to all.

The swinging Sixties and Seventies

During the 1960s perfume became more affordable and people began to buy it as a regular treat. No longer were dressing tables assigned to just one signature scent; instead, a line-up of perfume bottles could grace their shelves. As holidays abroad became popular, duty-free shops also experienced a dramatic increase in perfume sales because the more expensive brands could be purchased at a tax-free price. Luxury favourites such as Chanel No 5, Joy and Miss Dior entered a popularity battle as cheaper but lovely perfumes from cosmetic houses such as Avon and Coty emerged onto the market.

In the 1970s, Yves Saint Laurent challenged the world of perfume with a completely new style of scent. Its groundbreaking, heady perfume Opium was marketed as a perfume to be worn only by the daring – and only during the evening. It became extremely popular very quickly, and other cosmetic houses were quick to follow suit with similar versions. Chanel launched Allure, an oriental-style fragrance; Estée Lauder followed with the spicy Cinnabar, while Yves Saint Laurent launched Poison.

In direct contrast, a range of light, fresh, daytime perfumes were also created for those not bold enough to wear the more powerful, heady styles. Lighter blends such as Nina Ricci's L'Air du Temps, Lancôme's O de Lancôme, Estée Lauder's White Linen, Issey Miyake's L'Eau D'Issey, Calvin Klein's Eternity and Cacharel's Anaïs Anaïs filled the lighter perfume void.

As perfume challenges continued, many more fragrances were brought onto the market – which meant that perfume was no longer the reserve of the rich and discerning. Schoolgirls could buy it with their pocket money. In fact, Charlie! by Revlon probably dominated every bus during (and after!) a school journey.

Advertising and celebrity endorsement

In order to get their products noticed, perfume houses engaged in expensive advertising campaigns designed to gain maximum exposure and attention. Small samples of perfumes were given away with magazines, accompanied by big, glossy colour photos that encouraged readers to aspire to certain lifestyles by wearing that particular fragrance. The idea of using celebrities to endorse a particular perfume quickly became fashionable. Today, linking a scent with the lifestyle of a film or pop star has become one of most successful ways of advertising perfume in history.

Perfumes for men

Yet even this wasn't enough for the perfume houses – nor, it seems, for consumers. Not content with producing perfumes for a predominately female market, the 1980s saw a huge shift towards creating fragrances for men. New, trendy Eighties men sought scents with 'masculine appeal', and perfumes with names such as Rodeo, Adidas, Arrogance, Gambler and Lamborghini were big hits.

'Perfumes for Men' were rebranded as aftershave products, and the perfume houses went crazy harnessing this new, lucrative market. Guy Laroche's immensely popular Drakkar Noir was an instant success, and it remains a top-seller today. Needless to say, the other cosmetic houses wanted a share of the male market and quickly launched their own range of men's aftershaves, with brands such as the ever-popular Aramis (owned by Estée Lauder) and Aramis Devin.

Unisex scents

Although not entirely new (centuries ago all perfumes were unisex), perfume houses also began to introduce scents aimed at both male and female perfume-wearers. Clarins' L'Eau Dynamissante and Calvin Klein's CK One were the first market leaders in the unisex revival. Because neither 'perfume' nor 'aftershave' seemed to be appropriate labels for this niche market, brands like these were dubbed 'body splashes'.

PERFUMES TODAY

Far from remaining complacent, perfume design and creation today is still a big adventure. I am certain that, in our lifetime, we will see new and innovative perfumed concoctions coming onto the market: for instance, perfumes that react with our senses and provoke different behavioural responses.

Innovative perfumes

One such fragrance already causing quite a stir is Molecule 01, developed by Escentric Molecules. Created using only perfumers' alcohol and a single aroma-chemical designed to mesh with the wearer's natural pheromones, the scent becomes individual to the wearer because the pheromones and the aroma-chemical form a uniquely aromatic bond. But it doesn't stop there; when human pheromones are engaged in this way, they become 'interested' in what is going on; this results in not just a fragrance, but a unique feeling, too. And since the perfume can be smelled on you by others, it is said to have an effect on their emotions as well.

Anti-perfumes

Another development has its roots, believe it or not, in the very quirky aroma of Stilton cheese. Eau de Stilton (seriously) is a blend of herbaceous aromas, including clary sage, yarrow and angelica seed. It is earthy, yet fruity – but I'm still not convinced I would wear it. It does, however, make a bold statement; it's daring and individual and certainly enables the wearer to break free from the perfume norm.

Following the proclamation of individuality come the 'anti-perfumes', two of which received massive interest when they were launched at London's Harvey Nichols department store. The first, Odeur 71, by Comme des Garçons, conjures up the aroma of 'dust on a hot light bulb, salty taste of battery, warm photocopier toner and fresh pencil shavings', while the other, Odeur 53, also from Comme des Garçons, is described as 'flaming rock, washing drying in the wind, flash of metal and nail polish'. Both are fascinating aromas and certainly wearable for those who want something different.

So you can see, in terms of perfume developments, from time immemorial to the present day, pretty much anything goes! You can't go wrong, because you are certain to end up with a blend that somebody will wear. By the time you've finished reading *Make Your Own Perfume*, you'll be equipped with the information, skills and knowledge you need to create the most stunning, breathtakingly beautiful perfumes that you and everyone you know will want to wear.

CHAPTER 1

Tools of the Trade

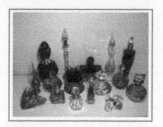

Very little specialist equipment is needed to make a range of perfumed products, and you will probably already have most of what is needed in your kitchen. However, be aware that perfume oils are very concentrated; once used for blending, your everyday bowls and jugs may be tainted with the taste of perfume. It is therefore recommended that you invest in a few specific utensils and pieces of equipment so that your perfume-making becomes a more pleasurable and easy experience.

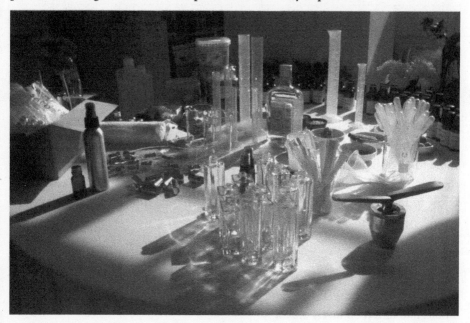

THE PERFUMER'S TOOLBOX

When starting to blend your own perfumes, you can make your job a little easier (and more enjoyable) by having different oils available to use. While a wide range of oils gives you choice and flexibility, even starting with just a few reliable, trusty oils will give you scope for experimenting without denting your budget too badly. Once you gain confidence, you may want to invest in more oils. The bigger selection of oils you have available, the more you can experiment, and the more varied your finished perfumes will be. I can't emphasise enough how beneficial and exciting it is to have a wealth of different perfume oils to choose from, but I also appreciate that the initial outlay can be expensive.

For that reason, I recommend the following 20 oils as a good starting point for your perfume toolbox. They will help you to structure a range of well-balanced, wonderfully aromatic perfumes and enable you to start making a range of structured perfumes suitable for men and women while keeping your costs at a reasonable level.

Top 20 'Must-have' Oils

Top Notes	Middle Notes	Base Notes
Bergamot (fruity)	Gardenia (floral)	Benzoin (oriental, sweet)
Clove (oriental, spicy)	Juniper Berry (green/woody)	Frankincense (oriental, spicy)
Lemon (fruity)	Mango (fruity)	Jasmine (floral)
Neroli (fruity/floral)	Bay (green)	Patchouli (woody)
Orange (fruity)	Tobacco Leaf (green)	Tonka Bean (oriental, sweet)
Petitgrain (fruity/woody)	Plum (fruity)	Rosewood (woody)
	Rose (floral)	Ylang-ylang (floral)

Dilutants

As well as having the oils with which to create your perfume blend, you will need some form of liquid in which to dilute them before they can be safely applied to the skin. We use either perfumers' alcohol or isopropyl myristate. *See* Chapter 7, 'How to Dilute Your Perfume Blends', for more information.

Cotton-wool pads

Use cotton-wool pads to create and test your blends. Once you have finished blending, you can put the pads in shoes, or place them in muslin/cotton bags to hang in your wardrobe, in the glove compartment of your car – anywhere that you would like to have a lovely smell!

Paper plates
Place the perfume-soaked cotton-wool pads on paper plates; that way, you can write on each plate exactly what is on each pad.

Pipettes
Use pipettes to dispense the oils from their bottles and for accurate measuring if your scales cannot weigh small quantities.

Mixing beakers and/or measuring cylinders
Mixing beakers have many uses. Use them to measure, mix and dilute your final perfume blends. Mixing beakers can be plastic or glass, whereas measuring beakers or cylinders tend to be plastic. Both beakers and cylinders should have clear markings on the side for measuring your ingredients.

Smelling sticks
Use smelling sticks to sample your perfume before you bottle it. You can also use them as samples to give to your friends.

Perfume bottles
You will need screwtop bottles in which to store your finished perfume creations. Ideally these should have a spray or roll-on attachment.

Stirring sticks
Used to stir your perfume oils and diluting ingredient. Wooden stirring sticks, the type you find in coffee bars for stirring cappuccinos, are ideal. Teaspoons are fine and do the same task, but make sure you clean them thoroughly, both before and after use. Glass stirring rods are also useful, as these can be used, washed and reused.

Glass jars with lid
Lidded glass jars can be used to hold cotton-wool perfume pads while they're given a chance to settle. Clean jam jars, baby-food jars and honey jars are ideal. Make sure these are thoroughly clean and odour-free by putting them through the dishwasher on a hot cycle, then allowing them to cool before use.

Heat source
If you plan to make solid perfume you will need a heat source for melting butters and waxes.

Double boiler and heatproof jug/bowl

Also used in making solid perfume. You will need a double boiler or similar in which to melt your ingredients.

Digital scales

Careful measuring and accuracy will ensure that one batch of perfume is identical to the next. While pipettes, measuring beakers and cylinders are useful, they aren't as accurate as digital scales. It is far easier to weigh 10g accurately than it is to measure 10ml.

Because you will be working in small quantities initially, weighing three or four drops of a perfume oil will be difficult unless you have very precise scales that can measure tiny quantities – such as scales that also measure precious metals like gold and silver. These aren't as hard to find as you might think; we bought our sets from eBay.

If you don't have scales to hand, then here is a useful, but not an absolutely accurate, guide: 25–30 drops of perfume oil is equal to 1g. This is fine as a rough rule of thumb, but be aware that this amount doesn't hold true for all oils. For example, patchouli essential oil is heavier than lemon; therefore 1g of patchouli will equal fewer drops than 1g of lemon oil.

You can also use the following chart as a rough measuring guide when creating your blends.

Perfume oil measuring chart

Number of Drops	Approximate Measurement	Approximate Volume	Approximate Weight
25–30 drops	¼ teaspoon	1ml	1g
50–60 drops	½ teaspoon	2.5ml	2.5g
125–150 drops	1 teaspoon	5ml	5g
375–450 drops	1 tablespoon	15ml	15g

Throughout *Make Your Own Perfume,* you'll find the quantity of perfumed products referred to in both ml and grams. For the purposes of this book, we consider these to be equal, so if a weight of 3g perfume oil is listed, you can use 3ml if that is your preferred way of measuring oils.

However, to follow the recipes exactly, you'll need to use either grams or ml and not combine the two measurements in the same recipe. If you do, you will have created your own variation of a perfume recipe – which is absolutely fine, but it will differ very slightly from the recipe in the book.

Notes/Log

The sooner you get into the habit of recording everything you do in terms of blending your perfume oils, the better. There is nothing more frustrating than creating a perfectly beautiful aroma and then forgetting not only which perfume oils you used, but the volumes of those perfume oils, too. Make your own copies of the Formulation Sheet below and use these to record the amount of oils and dilution solution you use each time.

FORMULATION SHEET

Date of formulation: 14th March

Name of formulation: Pink Heart

Blend of formulation:

Oils	Quantity
Sweet Orange essential oil	5 drops
Bergamot essential oil	9 drops
Juniper Berry essential oil	2 drops
Rose fragrance oil	11 drops
Tuberose fragrance oil	14 drops
Jasmine fragrance oil	5 drops
Patchouli essential oil	4 drops
Amber fragrance oil	10 drops
TOTAL BLEND	60 drops (2ml)
Diluted with perfumers' alcohol	38ml
TOTAL PERFUME (Eau de toilette) made	40ml

Protective clothing

Always wear a protective apron when working with oils and be aware that splashes can permanently mark your clothing. If you have long hair, you'll need something to tie it back with so that no stray hairs fall into your perfumed products. Since perfume oils are undiluted, we also advise wearing some thin rubber, vinyl or nitrile gloves to avoid any adverse skin reactions.

CHAPTER 2

A Sensible Approach to Health and Safety

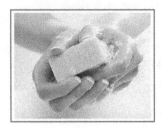

While it isn't compulsory to sterilise your equipment, you must ensure that it is clean, that your ingredients are stored properly so that they remain fresh and safe, and that your packaging is kept dust-free and spotless.

Keep your equipment clean

Before you use any utensil or equipment, make sure that it is clean and dust-free. Wipe it with a piece of kitchen paper or a clean cloth just to make sure. It is not necessary to sterilise your equipment, but if you want, you can use commercial sterilising solutions designed for baby bottles; full instructions are given on the back of the containers, and the solution is available from most chemists. Alternatively, immerse your equipment into boiling water for 15 minutes, then leave it to cool – but only do this if you're certain the equipment can withstand very high temperatures.

Remember to clean any kitchen work surfaces with a suitable kitchen cleaner both before and after creating your perfumed products.

Cleaning pipettes and beakers

Pipettes and beakers can be washed and reused. To clean pipettes, fill a bowl or jug with very hot water. Squeeze any remaining oil residue out of the pipette on to a tissue or similar, then draw in as much hot water as you can. Squeeze out this water into another container – not back into the bowl or jug. Repeat the process, drawing more clean hot water into the pipette until you're satisfied that all perfume residue has been removed. Finally, leave the pipette upright to drain and dry.

Handling perfume ingredients

The perfume oils mentioned throughout this book will either be a natural essential oil or a synthetic fragrance oil. All the perfume oils are undiluted potent compounds; they are too strong to be applied directly to your skin and will need diluting prior to use. For this reason you may wish to wear protective gloves. Do wash your hands after handling the bottles in any case, avoid direct skin contact with the undiluted oils, and avoid touching your face. Many oils are flammable and act as strong solvents. Eucalyptus oil, for example, can be used to remove glue from old stickers or to strip paint. As such, all oils should be handled carefully.

Eye exposure

If any of the ingredients accidentally splash into your eye, flush the affected eye immediately with copious amounts of MILK for at least 15 minutes. Seek medical advice if painful stinging or reddening symptoms persist.

Ingestion

Obviously, you should keep all perfume ingredients away from children and pets. Perfume oils have a wonderful scent, and some often smell like delicious food products. However, they are *not* edible, so never swallow or attempt to take the oils internally. If you do accidentally swallow any oils, rinse your mouth with MILK and seek medical attention immediately.

Spillage

Clean any spillage with an absorbent material such as kitchen roll. Remember to wear protective gloves while doing so, especially if the spillage is excessive.

Handling

Do not eat, drink or smoke when handling essential or fragrance oils. Respect good personal hygiene and wash your hands both before and after use. Avoid touching your face, especially your eyes and mouth, when you have handled oils. Always mix perfume oils with perfumers' alcohol or other appropriate diluting ingredient before applying them to you skin. Never apply diluted perfume oils to inflamed or broken skin, and do not use perfume oils undiluted on skin. If you're pregnant, or have any underlying illness, seek medical advice before handling or using essential oils.

Storage

Store all perfume ingredients in a cool, dry place, away from heat and direct sunlight. Store the ingredients in their original containers and make sure they are labelled so that the contents can be easily identified. Avoid contact with polished surfaces and plastic as the perfume oils may damage or stain the surface.

First use

Before using any of the finished perfumed products you make, you should consider carrying out a patch test. This involves placing a little of the finished perfumed product on the skin of the inner arm. If there is no redness, itchiness or adverse reaction to the product after 24 hours, then it is fine for you to use.

Cosmetic regulations

The perfumed products made in this book are for personal use only – they must not be sold commercially. If you intend to make and sell cosmetic products, your product formulation must be certified by a cosmetic chemist and conform to EU Cosmetic Regulations.

CHAPTER 3

Creating Your Perfume

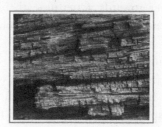

Creating a perfume is an adventure, and it is one that should never be skimped on or rushed. Before embarking on your perfume-making journey, you need to appreciate and understand several stages in order to guarantee a successful end product: a beautiful handmade perfume.

This may initially look like a lengthy and complicated exercise, but the process has been broken down into manageable segments, allowing you to understand and become familiar with the character, personality and nature of all the perfume ingredients and processes involved. Let's start by looking at the different fragrance families.

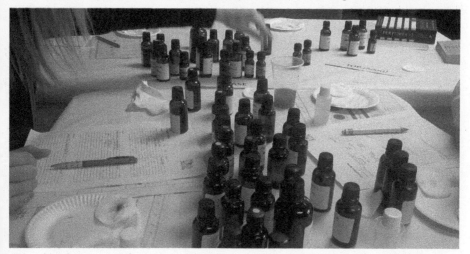

When blending your perfumes, you can make your job easier by having several different oils available to use.

FRAGRANCE FAMILIES

When purchasing a perfume, most of us stay within our comfort zone, selecting a scent from a fragrance group we recognise and know we're likely to get on with. Some of us may prefer sweet, floral perfumes while some choose light, fruity ones; the boldest may reach for the spicy, oriental fragrances. More often than not, however, we veer towards a perfume that is similar to what we've been used to whenever we make a selection. These groups or categories are called Fragrance Families.

Have a sniff of a perfume and try to describe exactly what you smell. Close your eyes and think about the first words that explain what you are experiencing. With some perfumes, this may be easy – words such as fruity, flowery, citrusy, musky, herbaceous, sweet, spicy, tart, sour, etc., spring to mind – but with others, it may be difficult to find the words that describe the overall aroma.

Over the centuries, perfumers have categorised aromas into different groups or 'families' according to their aroma type. Some families are further divided into subcategories. The main categories – or fragrance families to give them their proper name – are Floral, Fruity, Woody, Oriental and Green.

Perfume-making stages

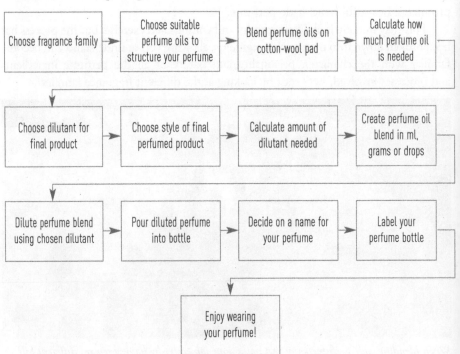

30

Floral fragrance family

Flowers are an obvious choice for assembling any smell, and floral perfumes are said to be romantic and symbolise love. From single-flower fragrances made from sweet but wonderful blooms such as rose, carnation, tuberose, lavender, gardenia, violet, jasmine, lilac and lily of the valley to bouquet combinations, floral perfumes will always be a popular choice.

A vast number of flower scents are used in the perfume industry. While two perfume houses may use the same combination of flowers, no two perfumes will smell exactly alike. Perfumes that fall into the floral category include:

- Lanvin's Arpège (lily of the valley, honeysuckle, hyacinth, lilac),
- Chanel No 5 (ylang-ylang, rose, jasmine, jonquil, iris, neroli, lily of the valley, mimosa),
- Issey Miyake's L'Eau D'Issey (pure white flowers, freesia, cyclamen, lily, tuberose, camellia),
- Paul Smith's Rose (self-explanatory),
- Jean Patou's Joy (roses, jasmine),
- Dior's Diorissimo (lily of the valley), and
- Lagerfeld's Chloé (tuberose).

Many of the floral smells in these perfumes are also mingled with gentle spices, ambers, musks and other secret ingredients, but the overall aroma is intensely floral.

Example Floral Blends

Creating your own blends gives you the ability to ensure that your favourite floral aromas form the predominant scents. Here are a few of our favourite blends. While some of them include aromas from the other fragrance families, the overall effect is abundantly floral.

Each perfume-blend recipe in the chart on the next page creates about 1ml of undiluted perfume, which must be diluted before using. Dilute this perfume blend with at least 9ml of perfumers' alcohol (for a fragrance) or 30ml jojoba oil (for a perfumed body oil) to make it suitable for use.

Directions Put 9–15ml perfumers' alcohol or 30ml jojoba oil in a mixing beaker. Add the required number of drops of perfume oils. Stir and decant into a perfume bottle.

Floral Perfume Blends

Rosy Pose	Vintage Dreams	In the Pink
16 drops Rose	15 drops Rose	18 drops Carnation
7 drops Vanilla	10 drops Jasmine	5 drops Rose
3 drops Ylang-ylang	2 drops Oakmoss	2 drops Clove
	1 drop Patchouli	
Midnight Moon	**Love Lore**	**Bouquet Spice**
9 drops Sweet Orange	6 drops Bergamot	12 drops Lavender
7 drops Neroli	5 drops Tuberose	4 drops Violet
7 drops Lily of the Valley	5 drops Gardenia	2 drops Clove
3 drops Ylang-ylang	5 drops Rose	2 drops Ylang-ylang
	3 drops Lily of the Valley	5 drops Honey
	4 drops Benzoin	

Fruity fragrance family

Fruit perfumes are said to be fresh, lively and uplifting. Luscious, fresh, exciting and almost edible, the fruity family includes aromas of mandarin, sweet or bitter orange, lemon, lime, grapefruit, tangerine, bergamot, apple, melon, peach, apricot, strawberry, passion-fruit, currants, pineapple, etc. They tend to have a citrusy freshness or a mellow, berry-like intensity that fill you with a delicious rush of mouth-watering surprises. Perfumes that fall into the fruity category include:

- Ralph Lauren's Lauren (pineapple),
- Calvin Klein's Escape (lychee, mandarin, apple, blackcurrant, plum, peach),
- Rochas' Femme (peaches, plums, apples, pears, apricots, citrus fruits),
- Lancôme's Ô De Lancôme (lemon, bergamot, tangerine), and
- Jo Malone's Pomegranate Noir (pomegranate, raspberry and plum).

Many of the fruity smells in these perfumes have been blended with spices, flowers and herbs to offset or intensify the juicy, fruit-like aromas that are bursting to climb out of the bottle.

Example Fruity Blends

Directions Put 9–15ml perfumers' alcohol or 30ml jojoba oil in a mixing beaker. Add the required number of drops of perfume oils. Stir and decant into a perfume bottle.

Fruity Perfume Blends

Berry Bang	Smoothie Too	Hot Tropical
10 drops Strawberry	15 drops Strawberry	3 drops Lemon
5 drops Watermelon	5 drops Mango	14 drops Orange
5 drops Mango	8 drops Vanilla	6 drops Mango
4 drops Lily of the Valley		3 drops Frangipani
4 drops Vanilla		3 drops Coconut
Carmen Miranda	**Very Berry**	**Moonshine**
5 drops Orange	7 drops Strawberry	4 drops Lemon
3 drops Lemon	4 drops Mango	4 drops Cucumber
2 drops Lime	5 drops Fig	4 drops Watermelon
3 drops Strawberry	4 drops Cucumber	8 drops Lavender
3 drops Plum	4 drops Benzoin	8 drops Vanilla
3 drops Passion Fruit	2 drops Patchouli	
2 drops Cherry		
2 drops Cucumber		
4 drops Honey		

Woody fragrance family

Woody perfumes are said to be lingering, heady and hypnotic. Sultry, smoky, earthy, peat-bog, damp, forest-type fragrances form the basis of this category. Aromas gathered from sap, resin, bark, leaves, ferns, roots and mosses combine to create classic fragrances. Oils of patchouli, vetiver, cedar, sandalwood, rosewood, pine, leather and tobacco all merge to create wonderful concentrations of secretive, smoky warmth.

While they are known for appearing in many aftershaves, woody aromas are not solely for the masculine market. They add an aromatic, woody undertone to any perfume designed for men, women or as a unisex scent. The woody family embraces mossy woods, dry woods and earthy woods. Perfumes that fall into the woody category include:

- Chanel No 19 (moss, fern, bracken, bark, sandalwood, cedar, sycamore),
- Lancôme's Magie Noir (sandalwood, .cedar), and
- Dior's Miss Dior (patchouli, oakmoss, galbanum).

Examples of woody male scents are:

- Aramis (sandalwood, oakmoss, leather),
- Geoffrey Beene's Grey Flannel (oakmoss, sandalwood), and
- Kenzo's Pour Homme (cedar, sandalwood, vetiver).

Many woody fragrances are blended with flowers, spices and herbs to soften the peaty dampness aspect of the woody aroma.

Example Woody Blends

Directions Put 9–15ml perfumers' alcohol or 30ml jojoba oil in a mixing beaker. Add the required number of drops of perfume oils. Stir and decant into a perfume bottle.

Woody Perfume Blends

Winter Witchery	Plush Folly Pamper	Burnished Coppice
15 drops Sandalwood	8 drops Bergamot	8 drops Mandarin
6 drops Geranium	8 drops Mandarin	4 drops Bay
3 drops Cedar	8 drops Juniper Berry	8 drops Rosewood
3 drops Patchouli	4 drops Patchouli	4 drops Patchouli
		1 drop Vetiver
Misty Moon	**Forbidden**	**Lost City**
4 drops Tobacco Leaf	2 drops Green Tea	2 drops Lime
2 drops Old Leather	2 drops Jasmine	2 drops Lemon
4 drops Rosewood	2 drops Labdanum	2 drops Mandarin
10 drops Oakmoss	1 drop Anise	12 drops Rosewood
4 drops Sandalwood	20 drops Sandalwood	4 drops Sandalwood
2 drops Patchouli		3 drops Patchouli
		1 drop Vetiver
		1 drop Ginger

Oriental fragrance family

Oriental perfumes are said to be provocative, lusty and seductive and with their trace of spicy, oriental bazaars, these fragrances are not for the faint-hearted! Said to be the strongest and longest-lasting of the fragrance categories, the oriental aromas include musk, resin, herbs, spices, amber and vanilla mixed with flowers of the Orient, including jasmine, rose and ylang-ylang. Astonishingly intense and exploding with sultry sweetness of aromas such as vanilla and jasmine, these perfumes tend to be worn in the evening rather than during the day.

Oriental aromas can be further split into sweet and spicy. The sweet aromas are typically vanilla, tonka bean, chocolate, honey, amber, benzoin and musk, while the spicy aromas are ginger, clove, cinnamon and black pepper. Some aromas either span both these sweet and spicy categories or don't fall into either camp. Aromas such as elemi, frankincense and myrrh are examples of these – they are neither sweet nor spicy. Perfumes that fall into the oriental category include:

- Guerlain's Shalimar (vanilla, conifer sap, sandalwood, opoponax, spices),
- Calvin Klein's Obsession (spice, oakmoss, coriander),
- Jean Paul Gaultier's Classique (amber, vanilla, wood),
- Dior's Poison (coriander, cinnamon, pepper, vanilla), and
- YSL's Opium (patchouli, balsam, benzoin, frankincense, ginger, cinnamon, coriander, cedarwood).

Many of these oriental perfumes have been balanced with multi-floral and citrus-fruit scents to lighten and adjust the cloying, syrupy headiness.

Note that there is an oriental subcategory called 'floriental', which is a combination of oriental and floral. It includes perfumes that are lighter than the heady orientals, yet spicier than the gently rich florals. These are suitable for daytime and evening wear and are perfect for those who are not quite brave enough to wear the true oriental perfumes!

Examples of perfumes sitting in the floriental *sub*category include Lancôme's Trésor (sandalwood, amber, musk, vanilla, lilac, iris, heliotrope, lily of the valley, violet) and Chanel's Allure (jasmine, vetiver, vanilla, magnolia, honeysuckle, rose, water lily).

Example Oriental Blends
Directions Put 9–15ml perfumers' alcohol or 30ml jojoba oil in a mixing beaker. Add the required number of drops of perfume oils. Stir and decant into a perfume bottle.

Oriental Perfume Blends

Ramji Spice	Lovelace	Outrageous
4 drops Tangerine	2 drops Mandarin	4 drops Mango
2 drops Lemon	4 drops Gardenia	5 drops Rose
12 drops Lavender	4 drops Clove	10 drops Pink Pepper
2 drops Ginger	8 drops Nutmeg	3 drops Patchouli
2 drops Clove	10 drops Amber	4 drops Honey
2 drops Cinnamon		2 drops Vanilla
Taj Nooram	**Midnight Desert**	**Renwick Island**
3 drops Orange	4 drops Neroli	5 drops Lime
3 drops Grapefruit	4 drops Jasmine	6 drops Mango
1 drop Peppermint	4 drops Carnation	1 drop Banana
4 drops Rose	4 drops Musk	2 drops Bay
2 drops Cinnamon	4 drops Sandalwood	4 drops Rose
2 drops Leather	4 drops Tonka Bean	2 drops Carnation
2 drops Patchouli	1 drop Chocolate	3 drops Coconut
6 drops Amber		3 drops Clove
4 drops Rosewood		1 drop Black Pepper

Green family fragrance

Green or green and fresh scents are fresh and youthful, vibrant and fun. These tend to be fresh fragrances such as grasses, juniper, aquatic, marine, pine, herbs and buds. If you like the smell of freshly cut grass, hedgerows, flower beds after the rain, crushed leaves, salty sea air and dewy wild flowers, this may be the category for you. Lush and verdant, these pure, fresh green smells include the following fragrances:

- Coty's Chypre (lavender, oakmoss, patchouli, clary sage, cypress, resin),
- Chanel's Allure (amber, hyacinth, ylang-ylang, cedar, sycamore, bark, bracken, moss, violet leaves),
- Estée Lauder's Alliage (jasmine, nutmeg, citrusy, green leaves, galbanum), and
- Balmain's Vent Vert (leaves, grasses, oakmoss, vetiver, bergamot, orange blossom, rose, galbanum, sandalwood, fern, lily of the valley, jonquil, hyacinth, spices).

Green perfumes are fortified with an assortment of florals, fruits, woods and orientals to enhance and intensify their green, fresh aroma.

Example Green Blends

Directions Put 9–15ml perfumers' alcohol or 30ml jojoba oil in a mixing beaker. Add the required number of drops of perfume oils. Stir and decant into a perfume bottle.

Green Perfume Blends

Spring Fresh	Summer Green	Autumn Air
6 drops Lime	6 drops Bergamot	4 drops Orange
6 drops Champagne	6 drops Cucumber	6 drops Fig
3 drops Bamboo	2 drops Juniper Berry	6 drops Tobacco
6 drops Lily of the Valley	4 drops Champagne	4 drops Clary Sage
3 drops Clary Sage	6 drops Lavender	2 drops Old Leather
2 drops Vetiver	3 drops Patchouli	4 drops Galbanum
Winter Ice	**Ozone Fire**	**Green Daisy**
2 drops Gooseberry	4 drops Juniper	1 drop Mint
8 drops Bamboo	4 drops Cypress	14 drops Lily of the Valley
6 drops Lavender	8 drops Salty Sea Dog	3 drops Frangipani
8 drops Fig Leaf	1 drop Violet	8 drops Green Apple
4 drops Oakmoss	3 drops Lavender	2 drops Nutmeg
	4 drops Amber	
	1 drop Cinnamon	
	2 drops Honey	

TO CONCLUDE...

- When choosing oils to use for designing your perfume, first decide what type of overall aroma you would like to achieve. The main fragrance families are floral, fruity, woody, oriental and green. While most people choose their favourite scent category, certain types of fragrances are suitable for different types of perfume. A lively, fruity perfume is more suitable for a light, daytime body spray, for example, whereas a sweet, haunting resinous aroma may be more suitable for a heavier, sultry night-time perfume.

PERFUME NOTES

All individual aromas are not only categorised into fragrance families, but they are also categorised into layers. These layers help you to structure your final perfume blend and enable the individual aromas to work in harmony with each other.

When you smell a perfume, your sense of smell is enjoying a special adventure. You don't smell just one aroma, but a chain of mini-aromas that eventually mingle to form an overall odour. The smell that hits your nose first is not necessarily the smell that lingers once the perfume has settled. This is due to the weight of the molecules of the individual oils that make up your perfume blend. The lightest molecule oils evaporate fastest and the heavier molecule oils evaporate slowest.

These layers are called top (or head) notes, middle (or heart) notes and base notes. They behave in very different ways and it is important to understand their behaviour, because it will have an impact on your final perfume blend.

Top notes

Top notes oils are the first aroma you smell when opening a bottle of perfume. They are the lightest in molecular structure and therefore evaporate into the air faster, travelling quickly up and out of the bottle (or off your skin if you're wearing the perfume) into the air and up your nose.

Top notes are typically stimulating and energising. They help make the perfume feel light and fresh. They play an important role in a perfume as they form the instant first impression of the fragrance. Top notes evaporate quickly, usually taking between five and 20 minutes to disappear. If you were to wear a perfume made up of only top notes the aroma would not be apparent for very long.

Top notes are usually derived from citrus fruits and are characterised by their sharp, tangy, stimulating aroma. Lemon is the lightest of all the oils and forms the first of the top notes, quickly followed by grapefruit and lime.

Fruits such as strawberry, blackcurrant, peach, mango, cherry and plum are heavier than the citrus fruits, and while you can include them in the top-note category, they tend to last a little longer than the lively top notes. These fruits are often labelled in the middle-note category, but may also be referred to as top to middle notes. If they take longer than 15–20 minutes to evaporate, then they are considered middle notes.

Middle notes

Middle notes usually form the main body of the perfume blend and define its character. As soon as your sense of smell has registered and recognised the top notes, the middle notes start to emerge, immediately changing the aroma your olfactory senses are experiencing.

Middle notes are usually obtained from flowers and herbs and are characterised by their strong, potent yet gentle and often soothing aroma. They can be invigorating, but they are not as lively or as refreshing as top notes. Middle notes typically take between 15–60 minutes to evaporate. Examples of middle notes are lavender, geranium, frangipani, rosemary, bay, basil and cucumber.

Heavier, richer, more heady floral aromas such as jasmine and ylang-ylang tend to be placed in the base-note category. Rose tends to be categorised as a middle-to-base note.

Base notes

Base notes are the big boys of perfume! They are the heaviest, and therefore hang around the longest, helping your perfume blend to last a long time.

Base notes are big, bold, rich and full-bodied. They are the last to emerge from the perfume but when they eventually make their appearance, they certainly make their presence known. Base notes finish off the perfume, influencing the aroma that lingers even after you've left the room. The final phase of the perfume, once all the individual scents have made their appearance and united in a glorious combination, is called the dry-down period. Because of the base notes' heavy molecular structure, it can take anything from one hour to several hours for a perfume to evaporate.

Base notes tend to come from the saps and resins, woods and syrups, beans and roots. They can be spicy, pungent, sweet or woody. Base notes are characterised by their almost intoxicating, soporific, relaxing, aphrodisiac, and long-lasting qualities. Examples of base notes include patchouli, sandalwood, vanilla, tonka bean, frankincense, amber and chocolate.

Fixatives and anchors

As well as giving a perfume depth and longevity, base notes have another important task – they act as fixatives or anchors for the notes that evaporate quickly. What this means is that, when blended with base notes, tops notes such as lemon or bergamot will not disappear so quickly. This is an extremely useful tool to use when creating your perfume blends.

If you want a perfume to smell predominantly of lemons and bergamot but want to ensure that the scent will last longer than 20 minutes, you need to structure your perfume so that it is top-heavy with citrus fruit notes, but also includes base notes such as benzoin or patchouli to give it depth and longevity. Get the balance just right and the overall sense of the perfume will be light, fresh citrus fruit notes with an interesting twist that keeps the perfume hanging around for a few hours.

Blending the same oils but in different proportions can produce perfumes that behave and smell quite different. As you can see, the perfume blends in the chart below all use the same individual aromas. However, the proportion of the aromas differs in each blend, and this causes the resulting perfume to smell and behave differently from its neighbour due to the top, middle and base note balance being readdressed in each one.

Blending chart

Blend One	Blend Two	Blend Three
Quick Citrus Rush	Steady Citrus	Forever Citrus!
33 drops Lemon	23 drops Lemon	20 drops Lemon
17 drops Bergamot	12 drops Bergamot	17 drops Bergamot
8 drops Lavender	23 drops Lavender	11 drops Lavender
2 drops Benzoin	4 drops Benzoin	8 drops Benzoin

Quick Citrus Rush

From the blends above, you can see that Blend One, 'Quick Citrus Rush', would be a very fresh, lively perfume. The sharp, tangy lemon and the uplifting bergamot make for an instantly refreshing aroma. As your nose adjusts to the citrus-fruit duo the fresh aroma of lavender wafts in. The citrusy notes enhance the sharper edge of the lavender, giving an overall effect of a zesty, almost spicy aroma. The benzoin, while strong and intense, is detectable but not overpowering, causing a sweet, almost balsamic dry-down.

Steady Citrus

Blend Two, Steady Citrus, has fewer citrus notes but still has the initial fresh, lively impact. This time as your nose adjusts to the citrus notes, the lavender wades rather than wafts in because it has been included at a much higher proportion. Rather than take on the sharper citrusy characteristics, it is the lavender that owns this perfume, reducing the citrus notes to a quiet subtle presence. This allows the lavender to work as an invigorating, herbaceous element that gradually yields to balsamic undertones.

Forever Citrus!

Blend Three, Forever Citrus!, still has the fresh introduction of citrus-fruit scents to create a lively, fresh first impression. This quickly gives way to a calming herbaceous hint of lavender that allows the benzoin plenty of time to emerge triumphant, giving the perfume a soft, sweet, warm, balsamic finish.

CHARACTERISTICS OF PERFUME NOTES

Top/Head Notes	Middle/Heart Notes	Base Notes
Typically from citrus fruit	Typically from flowers and herbs	Typically from woods, resins, syrups and beans
Sharp and fresh, light and appealing, they are the first impression of the perfume	Flowery, gentle yet potent, make up the heart of the perfume	Heavy and with the greatest molecular weight. Spicy, rich and heady, base notes round off the perfume's aroma
Quick smell, short-lived, disappear quickly	A little slower to emerge and a little slower to disappear	Last to emerge, big presence, hang around and linger
Evaporates quickly, usually between 5–30 minutes	Evaporation is moderately quick: between 15 minutes to an hour	Evaporate slowly over a number of hours and help slow the evaporation of the other notes
Typically stimulating and uplifting	Typically balancing and calming	Typically relaxing and aphrodisiac

Linear perfumes

A perfume will most likely contain oils from a range of top, middle and base notes. Any perfume that doesn't have the traditional top, middle and base notes is described as 'linear'. While linear perfumes can still be as appealing as a top, middle and base note structured perfume, they may not be as refreshing or long-lasting.

Fragrance note confusion

If using the internet to research whether a fragrance is classified as a top note or a middle note, you may be baffled to find that it is listed under different categories, depending on which website you visit. Don't worry or let this confuse you; the decision really boils down to the behaviour of the oil and how quickly it evaporates.

Let's take ylang-ylang as an example. Ylang-ylang is a flower and therefore the obvious category for it is as a middle note, because these typically are flowers and herbs. Yet ylang-ylang is a very heady smell – rather like a lily. It is a heavy oil with a heady aroma and takes longer than an hour to evaporate. So it behaves as if it's a base note and therefore correctly belongs in that category.

As with all perfume creations, it's a question of experimenting. Find out how ylang-ylang and other oils behave in your formula and how quickly they evaporate.

While the top, middle and base note chart displayed here is useful as a guide to help you select balanced aromas, you can have an enormous amount of fun playing around to decide on the final structure of your perfume.

Where an aroma is listed as top (to middle), this means that while it has most of the characteristics of a top note, it may have a tendency to last a little longer, taking it towards the middle-note evaporation time frame. The same applies to aromas listed as base (to middle) – these aromas have a heady, rich, spicy or syrupy presence but have a slightly shorter evaporation window.

Note categorisations

Top/head note	Middle/heart note		Base note
Anise	Bamboo	Hyacinth (to base)	Amber
Apple	Basil	Juniper berry	Benzoin
Bergamot	Bay	Lavender	Cedar
Clove (to middle)	Blackcurrant (to top)	Lilac (to base)	Chocolate
Eucalyptus	Chamomile	Lily of the Valley	Coffee
Galbanum	Champagne	Mango (to top)	Frankincense
Ginger	Cherry	May Chang (to top)	Gardenia (to middle)
Grapefruit	Cinnamon	Palmarosa	Honey
Lemon	Clary Sage	Peach (to top)	Jasmine
Mandarin	Coconut	Plum (to top)	Labdanum
Neroli	Coriander (to top)	Rosemary	Leather
Orange	Cucumber	Salty Sea Dog	Myrrh
Peppermint	Fig	Strawberry	Oakmoss
Pepper	Frangipani	Tea	Patchouli
Petitgrain	Geranium	Tobacco Leaf	Rose (to middle)
Pomegranate (to middle)	Grass	Violet	Rosewood
			Sandalwood
			Tonka Bean
			Tuberose
			Vanilla
			Vetiver
			Ylang-ylang

BALANCING PERFUME BLENDS

It doesn't matter what ratio of top, middle and base notes you include in your final perfume so long as you have achieved what you set out to achieve. Your perfume can have a fruity presence that is fixed with a base note, which makes it last longer. Alternatively, you may want a citrusy introduction that then gives way to a big, powerful floral bouquet. There again, you may not want any citrusy note at all!

There is no right or wrong way of choosing your individual blends; you simply have to try out many variations of the blended aromas until you find a combination that seems perfect to your nose.

Blending techniques

Here are some techniques you can use to get the best from your perfume blend.

Using a fixative As you now know, top notes evaporate quickly, middle notes evaporate fairly fast but not as quickly as the top notes. The secret is to get the balance right and to include a base-note fixative that locks the smell down without overpowering it. If in doubt, work on six to eight times as much top note to base note. This will yield a lively perfume with a hint of base note, but still enable the top note to hang around for longer than it would without a base note to fix it.

Allow a settling period Another factor to work with is the knowledge that as top and middle notes evaporate, your perfume will change its smell. When creating a perfume, it's important to leave your sample blend for at least two hours at room temperature in order to evaluate its final aroma. This will allow the top and middle notes to flee or to be locked in – whichever you have planned for.

Add a touch of spice! Many of the fruity smells in perfumes can be blended with spices, flowers and herbs to offset or intensify those juicy, fruit-like aromas bursting to climb out of the bottle. This is a clever move, because the spicy base notes also help the top notes last longer because they act as a fixative. Think of the principle of adding pepper to your food. It isn't to make your food taste of pepper, but rather to season and bring out the food's flavour. The same applies to perfume-making. Experiment by adding add a little spice, such as ginger, black pepper or clove, to intensify and bring out the aroma of other fragrances.

Three very different but balanced perfumes

Cherry Lola	More Flora	Secret Ambrosia
2 parts Orange	1 part Neroli	1 part Bergamot
2 parts Bergamot	1 part Bergamot	1 part Gardenia
3 parts Cherry	2 parts Frangipani	1 part Rose
2 part Mango	2 parts Rose	1 part Bay
1 part Benzoin	2 parts Tuberose	2 parts Benzoin
	2 parts Rosewood	2 parts Honey
		2 parts Amber

The perfumes described above are all very different, even though they all have at least bergamot in common.

Cherry Lola

Cherry Lola is a light, fresh, daytime perfume. It has four citrusy parts, two of orange and two of bergamot, giving it a very obvious, fresh, citrusy introduction. Because orange and bergamot are light and evaporate quickly, the aroma will soon change to embrace the cherry and mango. Cherry and mango are middle notes, so add a longer-lasting layer of sweet fruit. Benzoin is both a base note and a fixative. It is sweet, warm and syrupy, adding to the perfume's depth. Benzoin takes over an hour to evaporate, so it gives this light, fruity perfume the ability to hang around for a while.

More Flora

More Flora also commences with citrus-fruit notes – but this time we have neroli teaming up with the bergamot. Neroli is the aroma extracted from orange blossom, so while it is citrusy, it is also floral, making it a perfect perfume ingredient. The top notes move over to allow the floral middle notes to take their place, and the mixture of frangipani, rose and tuberose form the biggest part of this perfume. To give this perfume a further floral twist and to ensure it has a base note to hang onto the smell, rosewood acts as the base note. Rosewood is an aromatic wood and, rather like the neroli offering a citrusy-floral tone, rosewood offers a woody-floral aspect, which rounds this perfume off beautifully.

Secret Ambrosia

The third perfume, Secret Ambrosia, is the most immediately obvious scent – it hangs around even after the wearer has left the room. Again, it is introduced by bergamot, but as this is the only top note, this perfume is slow to emerge. It won't rush in and surprise you; instead, it takes its time, luring you in to enjoy its fragrance.

The floral notes of gardenia and rose are given a slightly herbaceous edge by pairing them with bay. But the really interesting part of this perfume wades in after the florals, ensuring that it leaves a positively oozing sweet, syrupy aroma of honey, benzoin and amber. This fragrance is not for the shy and retiring; it's bold and makes a statement and leaves an impression not to be forgotten in a hurry.

Each of these perfumes would take you on an aroma adventure. From the moment your sense of smell detects the citrusy notes, meanders through to the florals, herbs and richer fruits and finally on to the sensuous lingering base notes with their woody, syrupy or honied contribution, your olfactory glands will enjoy the ensemble of different aromas, delighting you every step of the way!

TO CONCLUDE...

- Structuring your perfume using a balance of top, middle and/or base notes is key to giving it character, depth, layers and longevity.
- Erratic top notes can be tamed and harnessed by carefully balancing them with more dependable, robust base notes.
- The interesting character of a perfume is determined by the layers of notes used.
- The more interesting the perfume, the more memorable it will be.

CHAPTER 4

Natural versus Synthetic

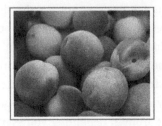

In your perusal of the perfume counters and when reading the perfume advertisements, you may have occasionally (very occasionally) come across a perfume promoting itself as being 'natural'. So what does 'natural' mean here and why aren't all perfumes natural?

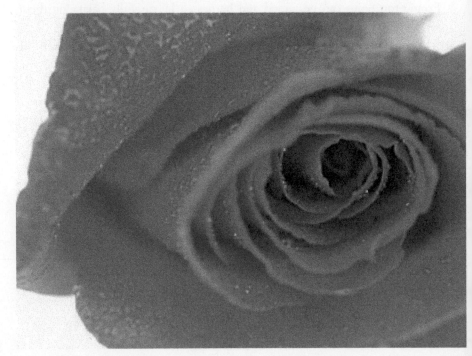

NATURAL PERFUMES

A perfume made from natural ingredients will use a blend of essential oils. Essential oils are extracted from plants and have a very strong, potent aroma. They are widely used in many luxury cosmetic products and form the basis of aromatherapy.

What is an essential oil?

Essential oils are plant oils that are volatile, meaning they are able to evaporate. Because they can evaporate, they are able to have an aroma – unlike other oils such as olive oil, sunflower oil and avocado oil. As essential oils evaporate, their molecules float into the air, around the room and up our noses!

Essential oil plant material

Many plants can yield an essential oil, but some plants lack the ability to produce an aroma that can be captured in an oil. Essential oils can extracted from different parts of the plant, such as from the petals, leaves, wood, seeds, bark, roots and stems. Typical essential oils include those extracted from:

- *Flowers* Rose, Jasmine, Geranium, Lavender, Ylang-ylang, Neroli (Orange Blossom)
- *Leaves/Grasses* Basil, Bay, Thyme, Rosemary, Lemon Grass, Vetiver
- *Fruit Peel* Orange, Lemon, Grapefruit, Lime, Mandarin, Bergamot
- *Seeds* Almond, Celery, Coriander, Black Pepper, Carrot Seed
- *Berry* Juniper, Pimento
- *Wood* Cedar, Sandalwood, Rosewood, Ho Wood
- *Bark* Cinnamon, Ravensara
- *Roots* Orris, Ginger
- *Resin* Frankincense, Myrrh, Benzoin
- *Moss* Oakmoss

Occasionally one plant will yield more than one aroma, each from a different part of that plant. An example of this is the orange tree. The blossom of the orange tree produces neroli, the pressed rind of the orange produces orange oil, and the unripe orange fruit, twigs and leaves produce petitgrain.

Essential oil extraction methods

The method chosen to extract essential oils depends on how well an oil reacts to heat and the volume of it likely to be produced. Extracting some oils requires vast amounts of plants for just a few kilos. For example, about 30 rose heads yields 1 drop of rose oil.

Different methods of extraction have been established according to the behaviour of various plants when exposed to heat, and to maximise the yield of oil. Since so many labour-intensive processes are involved, the cost of essential oils can be very expensive. Plant crops are vulnerable not only to heat, but to bad weather conditions, variable climate and environmental damage. The price of some essential oils can change on a regular basis, making the market unpredictable and unsteady.

Steam distillation The more common method of extracting oil from a plant is via steam distillation. Oils such as rose, neroli, rosemary and lavender are extracted in this way. The plant parts are immersed in boiling water to enable them to release their natural aroma into the steam. When the steam and oil vapour are cooled, the steam reverts to water while the oil forms droplets on it. The oil and the water are now separated. The oil is the essential oil and the water is the hydrolat (also known as floral water).

Enfleurage Some plants don't respond well to heat. Jasmine is one such example, since it loses its heat in the warmth of the sun and is at its most aromatic early in the morning. Using steam distillation on jasmine destroys its beautiful aroma, so a different method is used to extract its aromatic oil. To extract delicate aromas such as jasmine, a sheet of glass is spread with fat (usually a soft coconut oil) and the flower petals are laid on the fat. Another sheet of fatty glass is then laid on top, creating a 'sandwich' of fat and petals. During a 12-week period, the petals are changed regularly until the fat has absorbed the aroma of jasmine from the petals. The fat is then washed with alcohol, allowing the scented oil to be separated from the solid fat.

Solvent extraction This is another method that is used for plant material that is sensitive to heat. A solvent is passed over the plant material several times; each time it absorbs some of the aroma. The solvent is then washed away, leaving an aromatic waxy substance known as a concrete. Plants that are extracted using this method include violet and hyacinth. If the solvent extraction had been performed on a resinous plant such as benzoin, the waxy substance would be called a resinoid instead of a concrete.

Absolutes An absolute is made by dissolving the concrete in an alcohol to liquefy any remaining fats or waxes. The alcohol is then distilled within a vacuum to remove any alcohol residue, leaving behind a very concentrated form of the original fragrance. This concentrated form is quite intense and has to be diluted fully before it can be used safely on the skin.

Expression The rinds of fruits such as orange, grapefruit, lemon, lime and tangerines can be squeezed and pressed until the oil oozes from the rind. This oil is then collected and forms the essential oil.

What is a fragrance oil?

A fragrance oil is a man-made artificial oil made to smell the same as its natural equivalent. It is not natural, although it may contain some natural components. Since essential oils are susceptible to weather, climate and the environment, they can be unreliable in terms of availability and consistency. If a particular oil becomes unavailable or scarce, it can have a devastating impact on any perfume that relies on it as an integral ingredient.

Synthetic fragrance oils have revolutionised perfume-making because they have enabled literally thousands of smells to be made available, regardless of the climate and environment and at a reasonable cost compared to some of the rare and therefore expensive natural counterparts.

Allergic reactions

Some people may sneeze or have some other adverse reaction to perfume. They may claim that they are allergic to perfume – but because every perfume has a different structure, it is possible that they may in fact be allergic to some elements of certain perfumes but not all. Identifying which component is the allergen is made easier these days because manufacturers are required to list sensitisers on perfume labels.

Sadly, there are some people who steer clear of perfumed products entirely after having experienced a bad reaction somewhere along the line. It isn't necessarily the synthetic ingredients they are allergic to, however; essential oils are plant material and these also contain sensitisers.

International Fragrance Association

Fragrance oils sold for use in cosmetics have to conform to rigorous tests and regulations set out by the International Fragrance Association (IFRA), ensuring that, under normal use, fragrance oils are safe to go on the skin in cosmetic products and perfumes.

Interestingly, essential oils are not subject to the same degree of scrutiny. Since they have been used for years in traditional medicine and perfumery, further testing is currently deemed unnecessary because their reputation speaks for itself.

SYNTHETIC PERFUMES

Nature identical

The definition of nature identical is 'A substance that has been produced synthetically, not usually from a natural starting material, in order to produce a material that is identical to that naturally occurring in nature.' *(Source: DweckData)*

An example of a common synthetically produced nature-identical ingredient is farnesol, which is found in orange blossom (neroli), rose, jasmine and linden flowers, but can also be copied using synthetic, man-made materials. In both cases, the ingredients listed on the label would be the same.

The introduction of nature-identical synthetic products in perfume-making was one of the biggest changes in perfume history. At last, ridiculously expensive aromas such as jasmine or rose could be reproduced identically at considerably lower costs and in huge quantities that had a very long shelf life.

Let's take the beautiful essence of rose as an example. Rose is an integral ingredient in any perfumer's toolbox. Considering that it takes approximately 30 rose heads to create just one drop of rose essential oil, it is a mind-blowingly costly commodity. A 10ml bottle (approximately two teaspoons) costs in the region of £80, depending on the quality.

If you're fortunate enough to smell some pure rose essential oil you may be surprised – or even disappointed. The aroma is so intense, heady, strong, intoxicating and powerful that sometimes it is not initially detected as rose, and it is only as you're moving away from the bottle that the floral element is recognised.

A good rose fragrance oil will be everything that you want it to be. It will smell of roses, trigger all sorts of happy feelings, offer a powerful, heady intensity in keeping with a base note and at an affordable price. Fragrance oils should cost you in the region of £3–£5 per 10ml bottle, but buying larger quantities will allow you to take advantage of economies of scale.

Living flower technology

When smelling a rose, it is the 'head space' – the area just above the flower – that holds the aroma. Steam distillation will distil the rose head to obtain the rose oil, but this can be different in scent to the head-space aroma.

This gives perfumers a problem. How can we capture something that isn't tangible and then bottle it? Living flower technology is the answer.

Living flower technology enables the entrapment of a plant's aroma gases. With the help of glass containers, tubing, computers and cables, it is possible to capture floral scents without even picking a single flower.

The flowers are grown in a vacuum-glass container, which prevents the plant's aroma from escaping into the atmosphere. The fragrance of the growing flower are captured by connecting a vacuum tube that inhales the molecules of the plant's aroma gases. The gases are then siphoned off and the molecules separated so that the molecular structure of the gasses can be analysed. This enables the perfume chemist to synthesise a copy of the molecular structure and allows us to wear a perfume that will have an aroma identical to that of an unpicked flower.

Similar technology is used to determine the scent of a flower's fragrance at different stages of its life cycle. This living flower technology allows perfumers to create variations of the same flower's scent. For example, when a lily first opens, it has a fresh, green aroma. When it is completely open, it gives off a rich, heavier, more cloying scent. After 24 hours, the aroma is more intense and exotic. As with all flowers, as soon as the lily is picked, the process of decay sets in, so the sooner the flower petals can be squeezed, distilled or macerated, the less chance of the scent of decay becoming part of the perfume oil. In addition, living flower technology allows flowers that yield little or no oil to be used in perfume-making. Examples of these include freesias and orchids.

Synthetic ingredients work hard

Synthetic materials have a wider role to play than the simple creation of a glorious aroma. Their goal is to enable the perfume to perform better. They are designed to enhance the aroma, make the perfume have a longer shelf life, slow evaporation to allow the smells to last longer, moisturise our skin or carry out some other perfume-related duty. Whatever their role, synthetic ingredients transformed the perfume industry, and it is very rare these days to find a commercially manufactured perfume that is 100% natural.

NATURAL VERSUS SYNTHETIC

Which is better: natural or synthetic? This is a question I am often asked, and I have to say that, honestly, when it comes to perfume-making, it simply shouldn't matter. Perfume is worn for its breathtakingly beautiful, heart-warming, mood-lifting aroma. My nose and my olfactory nerves tell me what's good and what's not so good, and at that stage, they aren't even aware of what is natural and what isn't. Cost is a major factor. If I can wear a wonderful perfume that doesn't hurt my budget – well, then, that lifts my spirits, too!

No matter which route you choose – natural, synthetic or a combination of both – there are strict rules and regulations that govern the manufacture of the products. These regulations apply to the raw ingredients and also to the finished perfumed product, to ensure that they will be as skin-safe as is humanely possible. Just think of hay-fever sufferers who may sneeze and itch when walking past a vase of beautiful flowers. Natural as the flowers may be, they can still cause an allergic reaction.

When making perfume it is likely that you will use a combination of both essential oils and fragrance oils. If you decide to make only natural perfumes you will limit the choice of ingredients available to you – and certainly bump up the price of your raw ingredients.

Natural blends

The blends described here are made with easily achievable, affordable natural essential oils. Blend them with a dilutant such as perfumers' alcohol or isopropyl myristate using the following ratios:

- Eau de parfum: 6 parts alcohol/ipm to 1 part perfume blend
- Eau de toilette : 10 parts alcohol/ipm to 1 part perfume blend

Green Smiles	Warrior Earth	Back to Nature
4 parts Bergamot	1 part Lime	1 part Orange
2 parts Grapefruit	1 part Eucalyptus	1 part Neroli
1 part Rosemary	4 parts Lavender	1 part Juniper Berry
1 part Coriander	1 part Cedar	1 part Rosewood
1 part Rose Geranium	1 part Rosewood	2 parts Benzoin
1 part Vetiver	2 parts Patchouli	
	1 part Vetiver	

Synthetic Blends

The blends described here are made with easily obtainable, affordable fragrance oils. Blend them with a dilutant such as perfumers' alcohol or isopropyl myristate using the following ratios:

- Eau de parfum: 6 parts alcohol/ipm to 1 part perfume blend
- Eau de toilette: 10 parts alcohol/ipm to 1 part perfume blend

Pink Smiles	Fragile Earth	Back to Basics
4 parts Neroli	1 part Peach	1 part Pomegranate
2 parts Jasmine	1 part Plum	1 part Frangipani
1 part Rose	4 parts Fig Leaf	1 part Bamboo
1 part Gardenia	1 part Strawberry	1 part Grass
1 part Honey	1 part Sandalwood	1 part Salty Sea Dog
1 part Vanilla	2 parts Vanilla	
	1 part Tonka Bean	

Blends made with natural and synthetic ingredients

I have suggested fragrance oils either where the essential oil does not exist or where it may be too costly for use. Blend them with a dilutant such as perfumers' alcohol or isopropyl myristate using the following ratios:

- Eau de parfum: 6 parts alcohol/ipm to 1 part perfume blend
- Eau de toilette: 10 parts alcohol/ipm to 1 part perfume blend

Rainbow Smiles	Warrior Earth	Back to Black
4 parts Bergamot essential oil	1 part Bergamot essential oil	1 part Lime essential oil
3 parts Lemon essential oil	1 part Petitgrain essential oil	1 part Cherry fragrance oil
2 parts Mango fragrance oil	4 parts Lavender essential oil	1 part Plum fragrance oil
1 part Tuberose fragrance oil	1 part Oakmoss fragrance oil	1 part Fig fragrance oil
1 part Palmarosa essential oil	1 part Rosewood essential oil	2 parts Coffee fragrance oil
1 part Patchouli essential oil	2 parts Patchouli essential oil	
	1 part Benzoin essential oil	

CHAPTER 5

Aroma Oil Profiles

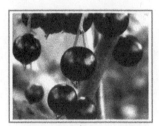

I am often asked which are the most useful and flexible essential and fragrance oils to include when making perfume. As I started compiling my 'staples' list, it grew very large, very quickly! It includes a selection of suitable aromatic essential and fragrance oils, all of which will give you the ability to build a variety of different perfumes. Use it as a guide when you start out. As you collect a portfolio of perfume oils, you'll add to this list, so let it guide you, but by no means let it be definitive. Choose other oils that you would like to experiment with, too. All the oils below come as a fragrance oil, but I've noted where a reasonably priced essential oil is also available.

Amber
Note: Base
Family: Oriental (sweet)
Amber will most likely be a fragrance oil unless you manage to secure some amber resin to infuse to make your own scented oil. Amber is a sweet, magical, soft fragrance that will help to fix your top notes. It blends well with both the sharper, fruity aromas and the softer, sweet aromas.

Anise
Note: Top
Family: Oriental (spicy)
Available as an essential oil, anise smells of liquorice and offers a rich, spicy aroma. Used in small proportions it adds an interesting twist to any perfume. Anise is an excellent aroma for offsetting an overly floral, sickly-sweet aroma.

Apple
Note: Top
Family: Green
While you can get both red- and green-apple fragrance oil, the latter is more useful. It adds an instant clean and fresh aroma and is a refreshing alternative to the usual citrus-fruit layer. Blends with other fruits, florals and sweeter honey and vanilla.

Bamboo
Note: Middle
Family: Green
A delightfully light, clean fragrance with ozone undertones. While bamboo is a member of the green fragrance family, it has a hint of oriental and a twist of citrus. Blends well with most aromas.

Basil
Note: Middle
Family: Green
Sweet, peppery and herbaceous, although I'm always slightly taken aback that this smells nothing like the basil plant on my kitchen window sill. Basil adds a spicy, green aromatic bite to any perfume. Available as an essential oil.

Bay
Note: Middle
Family: Green
I love the smell of bay leaves in cooking and the essential oil smells exactly as I would expect. West Indian bay is my favourite and I find it especially useful when formulating for a safe men's aftershave because it offers a trace of citrus, herbs and spice.

Benzoin
Note: Base
Family: Oriental (sweet)
Benzoin essential oil is a thick, viscous liquid that presents a medicinal, sweet aroma. It is soft and balsamic and blends with almost anything. Benzoin is used as a fixative for the lighter oils and is worthy of its place in ancient perfumery.

Blend benzoin with fruits, woods, orientals and greens and you will love the results. Blend it with the heady florals such as tuberose, jasmine and rose and you'll be delighted with your perfume blend. Benzoin must definitely form part of your perfume-making tool kit.

Bergamot
Note: Top
Family: Fruity
My all-time favourite for many reasons. Bergamot is a traditional perfume ingredient and I see no reason to change the course of history. Fruity, mildly spicy, radiant and uplifting, it blends with most other oils and gives a fresh, warm introduction to perfume. Available as an essential oil – and also a key ingredient in Earl Grey tea.

Blackcurrant
Note: Middle to Top
Family: Fruity
Not reminiscent of a syrupy drink, but more the aroma of the blackcurrant on the bush. Bud, leaves, fruit and stalks, a good blackcurrant fragrance oil will capture the entire aromatic plant and bottle it. Blackcurrant adds a delicately musky angle to any perfume and enables you to play around without overpowering the final perfume. It blends well with other fruits and woods.

Cedar
Note: Base
Family: Woody
Reminiscent of beehives and pencils, cedar is distilled from sawdust and wood shavings discarded in pencil production. Dry, soft and warm, the essential oils of both Virginian and atlas cedar are a perfect addition to men's aftershave. Blends beautifully with other woody notes and helps to control some of the more lively top notes.

Chamomile
Note: Middle
Family: Green
The straw-like grassiness of chamomile adds a dry, herbaceous softness to perfumes. Available as a slightly costly essential oil, you'd be forgiven for reaching for the fragrance oil instead. Blends well with greens and citrus, woods and spices.

Champagne
Note: Middle
Family: Green
Champagne fragrance oil brings a fizzing, fresh-grape aroma and wraps your perfumes in a perfectly feminine layer. Sparkling, exciting, fruity and fun – just what a light daytime perfume is crying out for. Blends with most florals, green and fruity notes, but can get a little lost in the woody base notes.

Cherry
Note: Middle
Family: Fruity
I have been searching for a cherry fragrance oil that doesn't immediately conjure up memories of children's medicine. A good cherry fragrance oil will be juicy, rich, fruity and sweet. Blends well with other red fruits and I find it gives an interesting sweetness to the grassy aromas.

Chocolate
Note: Base
Family: Oriental (sweet)
Find the right chocolate essential oil and you're in luck. The subtle scent of rich, dark, drooling chocolate can be the perfect finish for perfumes. Bittersweet, decadent, mouth-watering aromas work better and blend better than sweet, milky chocolate, but each to his or her own. I often add a tiny amount of chocolate – not for the chocolate aroma, but for the beautiful soft, rounded finish it gives a perfume.

Cinnamon
Note: Middle
Family: Oriental (spicy)
Cinnamon essential oil is steam-distilled from either the bark, the leaves or the root – each part of the plant yields a slightly different aroma. The piquant aroma makes an ideal ingredient in perfumes and adds a spicy warmth that is both powerful and tenacious. Cinnamon blends well with citrus, spicy orientals and woods. Use sparingly.

Clary Sage
Note: Middle
Family: Green
Essential oil of clary sage gives a sweet, nutty herbaceous aroma and blends well with all citrus oils.

Clove
Note: Top to Middle
Family: Oriental (spicy)
The entire clove tree is aromatic, resulting in two subtly different essential oils: clove bud and clove leaf. Clove leaf is less concentrated than the bud and often easier to work with in terms of intensity. The leaf oil is fresh and spicy, while the bud essential oil has more woody undertones.

This is a delightful oil to use in perfumes, the perfect alternative to a citrus introduction and it will help to boost a rose or carnation. Eugenol is a natural compound found in both the clove leaf and bud. It is also present in rose and carnation and forms part of the 'perfume building blocks' of these oils. Blending clove with rose or carnation helps to enhance the floral aroma. Clove blends beautifully with most florals. Use sparingly.

Coconut
Note: Middle
Family: Green
Coconut fragrance oil comes in different levels of aromatic sweetness, from the creamy piña colada to the fresh, 'just cracked the coconut open' aroma; I prefer the latter. Coconut imparts a delicate freshness, a tropical hint and a twist of holiday mood. Blends well with most other aromas.

Coffee
Note: Base
Family: Oriental (spicy)
Available as an essential oil, although this is quite difficult to find, so the fragrance oil is a more likely option. Rich, deep, freshly roasted coffee can give the most delicious twist to your blend. A simple blend of coffee and fresh citrus is surprisingly addictive.

Coriander
Note: Middle to top
Family: Green/Oriental
Fresh, light, lively, uplifting, peppery, sweet, woody – in fact, coriander will pretty much give you a whirlwind of different sensations, apart from floral and cloying sweetness. Use coriander essential oil to give a refreshing polish to your perfume.

Cucumber
Note: Middle
Family: Green
Who would have thought that cucumber fragrance oil could offer such a lovely aroma? Prettily floral with a hint of a summer's day, cucumber is a perfect addition to fresh, light floral perfumes. Blends well with fruits and florals.

Eucalyptus
Note: Top
Family: Green
Eucalyptus essential oil will enable your perfume to arrive exploding and bursting from the bottle – what a lively aroma! It is fresh, herbaceous and menthol-like and blends well with other herbs and flowers. It is an energetic top note so doesn't hang around long, giving the more mature aromas a chance to envelop you.

Fig
Note: Middle
Family: Green/Fruity
Fragrance oils of fig (the fruit) and fig leaf are completely different. Fruity fig will add a juicy, fruity layer that can soften zesty citrus and lighten rich berries, while fig leaf adds a fresh, spicy, surprisingly verdant tang. Both blend well with other aromas.

Frangipani
Note: Middle
Family: Floral
Lovely floral fragrance oil of frangipani instantly conjures up a summer breeze cooling the hot sun on your skin. Very feminine, very pretty and very lovely, frangipani blends well with other florals and is particularly good with aromatic woods and rich fruits.

Frankincense
Note: Base
Family: Oriental (spicy)
If you can afford the essential oil, then I encourage you to use this in preference to the fragrance-oil version. The deep, haunting, exotic aroma of frankincense has been utilised as a perfume ingredient for years. Used extensively in meditation, frankincense can have a soothing effect and impart a feeling of peace. Blends well with most other oils and will help to fix top notes.

Galbanum
Note: Top or Base
Family: Green/Woody
A hard-to-get-hold-of essential oil. You will more easily find this as a fragrance oil. Depending on from which part of the plant galbanum has been extracted, it will be either a rich, balsamic, resinous base note or a light, woody, soft top note that blends extremely well with other woods and greens.

Gardenia
Note: Base (to middle)
Family: Floral
Fragrance oil of gardenia is exquisite. It simply radiates with the aroma of fresh, white, clean, intoxicating florals and is delightful in both small and large proportions in your blend. Keep your perfume simple and just add a touch of rosewood or ylang-ylang, or add a complex mix of other florals, citrus, aromatic woods and resins – gardenia loves them all.

Geranium
Note: Middle
Family: Floral
While technically a flower, you could quite easily believe that essential oil of geranium also belongs in the green fragrance family, and the oil is in fact distilled from the leaves and stems of the aromatic bush. Geranium provides a bright, uplifting scent that won't overpower your perfume, making it a favourite in lighter florals – no intoxicating, headiness here. It blends well with most florals, fruits and woods. Another member of the geranium family is rose geranium, which offers a deeper, more rosy finish and helps to boost the floral aroma.

Ginger
Note: Top
Family: Oriental (spicy)
Spicy essential oil of ginger is distilled from ginger root. As a top note it is an initially lively and obvious smell that can run the risk of overpowering other top notes. In the right proportions it will work in synergy with orange, lemon and lime to offer a warm citrus aroma.

Ginger also blends with with florals, enabling you to create your own versions of ginger lily, ginger rose and similar. It likes to merge with the woody aromas as well to offer a spicy, stimulating undertone. Ginger fragrance oils capture the essence of gingerbread rather than the pungent spice and can create comforting, homely blends.

Grapefruit
Note: Top
Family: Fruity
Grapefruit is an extremely versatile essential oil. You can sharpen it with lime and lemon, encourage it to take on a spicy twist with lavender or geranium, or tame it with heavier florals such as gardenia, ylang-ylang or tuberose.

Grass
Note: Middle
Family: Green

From the smell of freshly mown lawn to dried, straw-like aromas, fragrance oil of grass can be found in many styles. Unmistakably green, fresh and, well, grassy (!), you can control and manipulate your perfume by adding woods (for a damper, more bog-like aroma) or flowers (for a summer's day meadow), grasses (for a walk in a field) or fruits (picnic in an orchard). As you can see, grass fragrance oil is a very flexible little friend and I'd definitely include this as a must-have.

Honey
Note: Base
Family: Oriental (sweet)

Oozing and dripping with a sweet charm, this delightful honeyed aroma adds a warm, sweet, smooth finish to any perfume. Do test a selection of honey fragrance oils to find the one you like best. True to its natural counterpart, honey can be composed from the nectar of flowers or herbs, garden flowers, hedgerow flowers and fruit-tree blossom, each of which will bring its own glorious flavour to the honey. Honey fragrance oils will vary, too.

Hyacinth
Note: Middle to base
Family: Floral

Although available as an essential oil, the price of a natural hyacinth oil is not for the faint-hearted! The good news is that a hyacinth fragrance oil will capture the deep, heady, floral-abundant aroma, making it the perfect floral ingredient for perfume. Hyacinth blends well with other florals and aromatic woods and can be subdued to a more woodland floral scent by blending it with patchouli or a mere smidgen of vetiver.

Jasmine
Note: Base
Family: Floral

Jasmine speaks for itself! A gloriously rich, sweet, powerful scent, jasmine makes a welcome and important appearance in many perfumes. Intensely floral, heady, sedating and sweet, jasmine is persistent and lingers unwaveringly. Natural jasmine oil will cost you dear, however, so I would reach out for the fragrance oil. However, do shop around, as the quality of jasmine fragrance oils can be a little hit-and-miss.

Jasmine blends well with all notes and is definitely one for your perfume toolbox. While not wishing you to have any feelings for jasmine other than one of wonder and enjoyment, I should tell you that jasmine contains a natural compound called indole. Indole gives a faecal-like undertone, imparting a cat-urine /-poo /decay type of smell. Don't despair! This doesn't overpower or mar the perfume and it is exactly this factor that makes jasmine so interesting – and luckily, so beautifully aromatic!

Juniper berry
Note: Middle
Family: Woody
Reminiscent of gin, this delightful essence conjures up an autumn walk. Distilled from the small berries of the juniper tree, this oil adds a light, woody, almost fruity layer to perfume. Blends well with other fruits and woods in particular, but also the lighter florals and grasses.

Labdanum
Note: Base
Family: Oriental (sweet)
Natural labdanum is the resinous discharge from the rock rose, a busy shrub. The fragrance oil is a good alternative and is less viscous than the essential oil. Labdanum adds a sweet, balsamic, amber-like tone to perfume and has the advantage of doubling as a fixative. It blends well with most other aromas, but is particularly good with citrus notes.

Lavender
Note: Middle
Family: Floral/Green
Lavender is such an interesting aroma. While we think of it as floral, it is also herbaceous, green, fresh and spicy. It can take on a different edge, depending on what it is blended with. Suitable for blending with delicate florals, sharper spices and rounded aromatic woods, lavender has something for every nose, as it blends with everything. Easily available and affordable in its essential-oil form.

Leather
Note: Base
Family: Oriental (spicy)
Leather might not be an aroma you'd necessarily think of adding to perfume, but please give it a try. In the fragrance-oil section, you will likely come across new

leather and old leather. New leather is more 'constant-sale-furniture outlet' aroma and will remind you of new leather sofas, belts and jackets, while old leather has that much-loved, settled in, comforting scent.

Dark and smoky, leather adds an interesting, almost bonfire-like twist to perfumes. It is the perfect ingredient in heavy, spicy, sultry, intense perfumes.

Lemon
Note: Top
Family: Fruity
Lemon always makes the first impression in a scent because it is the lightest of all the essential oils. Exciting, lively, fizzing and desperate to escape, it will rush at you like an excited child, demanding attention. Sadly, like that impetuous child, it soon loses interest and flees, leaving you to study the rest of the perfume.

Big fixative base notes will exert their powers and help to anchor the energetic lemon, ensuring that it hangs around and does its job properly – allowing the lovely citrus aroma to blend throughout the perfume, giving it longevity.

Lilac
Note: Middle to Base
Family: Floral
With its very short lifespan, lilac is always in short supply but in high demand, making it both difficult and expensive to obtain. However, the delicious fragrance oil equivalents are beautiful. Lilac is one of the most aromatic flowers and is popular with birds, bees, butterflies and perfumers! Blends well with other florals and soft juicy, sweet fruits.

Lily of the Valley
Note: Middle
Family: Floral
Such a pretty flower, such a gorgeous smell, such a vital perfume ingredient! Lily of the valley is notoriously difficult to capture as an essential oil, so do opt for the fragrance oil instead. Lily of the valley offers a deep, heady floral aroma cheekily edged with a little spice.

Mandarin
Note: Top
Family: Fruity
Less citric than sweet orange and with the aroma of a rind rather than juice, mandarin essential oil will bring a slightly bitter citrus scent to your perfume.

Refreshing without being tart or sour, it hangs around for longer than its other citrus cousins, and allows the middle notes to emerge through its fruity presence. Blends well with other citrus, woods and grasses.

Mango
Note: Middle to top
Family: Fruity
Mango fragrance oil makes a welcome addition to many perfumes. While it partners well with other fruits, it also softens the sharper, tangy aroma of citrus and blends it to a smoother, rounder almost creamy aroma. Mouth-wateringly beautiful, mango blends with florals, greens, fruits and sweet orientals making it a versatile perfume ingredient.

May Chang
Note: Middle to top
Family: Fruity
May chang essential oil is also known as *Litsea cubeba*. It is intensely lemony and will give a fresh citrus note to perfumes that lasts longer than the regular top-note citrus, which makes it an especially useful ingredient in perfume-making. May chang blends well with woods and citrus. It is also a more flexible alternative to Lemon Grass.

Myrrh
Note: Base
Family: Oriental (spicy)
Myrrh is a strong, powerful, spiritual scent that brings a spicy warmth to perfume. The essential oil of myrrh blends well with other spicy orientals such as frankincense, and heady florals such as jasmine.

Myrrh also helps to fix a perfume blend.

Neroli
Note: Top
Family: Floral
Neroli is extracted from the blossom of the bitter-orange tree. Given the fact that the tree is not in blossom for long and that the blossom doesn't yield much oil, neroli is an expensive essential oil. Fragrance oil copies are often very true to their natural counterparts and make a beautiful addition to perfumes. Neroli crosses the border of floral to fruity and you can detect a soft floral aroma in it, with a hint of citrus. It blends well with florals, citrus and orientals.

Oakmoss
Note: Base
Family: Woody

Natural oakmoss is obtained from a soft, mossy lichen that grows mainly on oak trees. While the moss itself doesn't have much of an aroma, once it has dried and matured it develops a woody, mossy, damp-woodland type of smell. Available as a moderately expensive essential oil, the fragrance oil copies are equally as aromatic and delicious.

Dark olive-green in colour, oakmoss not only adds a wonderful rounded, woody aroma, but it also acts as a fixative while adding a tinge of green to your final perfume blend. It blends well with most other aromas.

Orange
Note: Top
Family: Fruity

Orange essential oil is extracted by pressing the orange peel. Deliciously fruity, but softer than lemon and lime, orange adds a feeling of warmth, coziness and a hug to your perfume blend. One of the most reasonably priced essential oils and a useful addition to your perfume toolbox.

Orange blends well with all other aromas, especially other citrus, orientals and woods.

Palmarosa
Note: Middle
Family: Floral

Palmarosa is steam-distilled from a grass, which yields an aromatic floral oil. The aroma is sweet and rosy, which is why this oil is often used with other florals to boost a delicate, rosy aroma.

Palmarosa blends well with other florals and citrus.

Patchouli
Note: Base
Family: Woody

Patchouli essential oil is rich, syrupy, dark brown and viscous and adds a very pleasant balsamic, herbaceous, sweet, earthy aroma to any perfume blend. Patchouli will help to fix an aroma and is a popular lingering perfume ingredient. This is definitely one for the perfume toolbox.

Patchouli blends well with all other aromas.

Peach
Note: Middle to top
Family: Fruity

A good peach fragrance oil will add a mellow, mouth-watering sweetness to your perfume blend. Used as a soft, fruity note in many brand-name perfumes, peach conjures up images of hot, lazy summer days. It blends well with other fruits and florals.

Pepper
Note: Top
Family: Oriental (spicy)

Black pepper essential oil is distilled from the dried, crushed peppercorns. As in food, a touch of black pepper can help to enhance other aromas, and slightly larger doses can add a spicy, pungent, stimulating aroma.

Pink pepper fragrance oil has a sweet yet spicy aroma and adds an oriental edge to a perfume blend. It is not heavily spiced, nor will it linger, but it will give your perfume an enthusiastic introduction.

Blend black pepper with other orientals, woods and citrus tones. Pink pepper blends well with florals, fruit and sweet oriental notes.

Peppermint
Note: Top
Family: Oriental (spicy)

Peppermint is an interesting essential oil to use in a perfume. It is lively and exciting, and while it offers an interesting twist as a top note, it is short-lived and disappears quickly. Peppermint is cooling on the skin and is often an addition to a light, refreshing body spray. It blends quite well with green notes, orientals and woods.

Petitgrain
Note: Top
Family: Fruity/Woody

Petitgrain essential oil is distilled from unripe citrus fruit, leaves and twigs, producing an aroma that has both citrusy and woody tones. Used extensively in men's aftershave, it is not exclusively a male aroma and helps to tame fizzing-sherbet citrus, making it a softer, more mature aroma.

Petitgrain blends well with other citrus, woods and spicy orientals.

Plum

Note: Middle to top

Family: Fruity

Another mouth-watering, juicy fruit that adds a deliciously sweet, rich, intense layer to a perfume blend. Plum fragrance oil is velvety soft. It's more along the lines of stewed plum ready for a dollop of double cream than freshly picked from the top of a tree. Blend your plum fragrance oil with other soft fruits, florals and green notes.

Pomegranate

Note: Top to middle

Family: Fruity

Pomegranate is a trendy, popular fragrance oil, adding a slightly tart, sharp aroma that blends perfectly well with other fruits, woods and orientals.

Rose

Note: Base to middle

Family: Floral

The cost of the essential oil can make this prohibitive for use in perfumes, so find yourself a beautiful fragrance oil version. Rich, heady and yet light and summery, rose adds a rich, floral intensity to any perfume blend. Rose aromas typify romance as roses are a symbol of love. Suitable for use in perfumes, aftershaves and unisex blends, rose is one of the most useful aromas for your perfume toolbox. It blends well with all other aromas, but especially well with other florals and sweet orientals.

Rosemary

Note: Middle

Family: Green

Rosemary essential oil is initially more aniseed menthol than herbaceous but it will mellow to give your perfume blend a green, fresh scent. Use sparingly, though, as rosemary does like to shout over the other aromas and announce its presence. It blends well with other green notes, woods and citrus.

Rosewood

Note: Base

Family: Woody

Rosewood essential oil crosses the borders of floral and woody, offering a delightful blend of both. Its rosy aroma is refreshing and sweet, yet spicy and woody, too. It makes a wonderful addition to men's aftershave and can subdue a lively, top-heavy daytime perfume blend. Rosewood blends well with other woods and florals.

Salty Sea Dog
Note: Middle to top
Family: Green

The relatively new, fresh, ozone, aquatic notes make a welcome addition to perfumes. Check out any fragrance oil that has 'sea' or 'salt' in it until you find one that works for you. Other ozone, fresh 'sea air' type fragrances include oils aptly named Sea Cucumber, Marine Vitality, Ocean Breeze, Sea Tonic, Blue Lagoon and so forth, but my particular favourite is Salty Sea Dog fragrance oil. It captures that tang of salty air you get when walking along a beach on a brisk, windy day.

Revitalising and energising, this aroma adds a remarkably invigorating layer to a perfume blend. Salty Sea Dog blends well with citrus, other green notes and spicy orientals.

Sandalwood
Note: Base
Family: Woody

The true, original sandalwood essential oil (from the *Santalum album* tree) is a rich, woody, viscous oil that will make an enormous dent in your pocket because it is very expensive. The more affordable sandalwood (*Amyris balsamifera*) is not related to *Santalum album*, yet it offers a more affordable alternative. While similar in smell, it is not as rich, but has a softer, haunting woody fragrance. Sandalwood blends well with most other aromas, especially citrus and other woods. It is a popular perfume ingredient.

Strawberry
Note: Middle to top
Family: Fruity

Strawberry fragrance oils can be a little hit-and-miss. Some strawberry oils conjure up the aroma of sweet shops, while others bring images of strawberries and cream and summer picnics. The hardest aroma to capture is that of a freshly picked big, juicy strawberry about to be popped into your mouth. Strawberry fragrance oil blends well with other fruits, florals and sweet orientals.

Tea
Note: Middle
Family: Green

Clean, calming, refreshing and soothing, tea fragrance oil adds a delicate and interesting layer to perfume. Green tea and jasmine tea have a floral softness, white tea has an exciting fruity edge, while black tea brings a tangy depth. All the teas blend well with everything and can enhance any floral, fruity, green or spicy perfume blend.

Tobacco Leaf
Note: Middle
Family: Green
Please don't imagine that tobacco leaf fragrance oil smells like a big fat cigar. The aroma is fresh and green, and is the essence of the leaf growing on the plant weeks before it is picked, dried, crushed and rolled into something unhealthy.

Fresh, green tobacco leaf imparts a clean, verdant, uplifting aroma, infinitely suitable for lighter perfumes and body sprays. Tobacco leaf blends well with citrus, other greens and woods.

Tonka Bean
Note: Base
Family: Oriental (sweet)
A cross between the cocoa and vanilla beans, tonka bean fragrance oil presents a deliciously sweet, tenacious caramel aroma. Not as sweet or as overpowering as chocolate, nor as obvious or sturdy as coffee, tonka bean rounds off a perfume blend, leaving a sweet, delicate welcome aroma that lingers. Tonka bean blends well with sweet orientals, fruits and florals.

Tuberose
Note: Base
Family: Floral
Tuberose fragrance oil gives a heady, exotic, sweet floral scent worthy of any floral perfume. Intense, intoxicating and powerful on its own, tuberose blends well with other florals and can be lightened with green, fresh notes and citrus. That said, you can blend the sweet tuberose with other sweet notes such as vanilla and tonka bean and the result is delightful.

Vanilla
Note: Base
Family: Oriental (sweet)
Another extremely useful addition to your perfume toolbox, fragrance oil of vanilla will add a syrupy, creamy layer to perfume. Extensively used as a fixative, vanilla adds longevity to a perfume, helping it linger. It blends well with most aromas, but particularly so with other sweet and spicy orientals, making it a mainstay in oriental-family perfumes.

Vetiver
Note: Base
Family: Woody
Highly valued for its ability to fix and hold on to a perfume's aroma, vetiver is an old perfume ingredient. Interestingly, it adds an earthy, old, stale-wood aroma to a perfume blend, which can impart an interesting musty edge.

Vetiver essential oil is extracted from an Indian grass and is extremely strong when bottled, putting many new perfume-makers off. However, it is well worth the effort of persevering with this oil because it blends superbly, creating new and exciting aromas.

Blend vetiver with other woody aromas, but also with green notes. It mixes particularly well with jasmine, sandalwood, patchouli and oakmoss.

Violet
Note: Middle
Family: Floral
Violet fragrance oil is not your usual heady, intoxicating floral aroma, but more a spicy, lively, interesting scent with a big impact. It stubbornly refuses to disappear into a floral bouquet but loiters around the edge, reminding you that it is still there.

Violet is perfect for both male and female blends because it can be interpreted as a spicy floral rather than a sweet, cloying floral. Violet blends well with citrus, woods and spicy orientals.

Ylang-ylang
Note: Base
Family: Floral
Ylang-ylang translates into 'flower of flowers', and at last makes an affordable essential oil that brings an abundantly glorious, rich, hypnotic, heady floral aroma. Ylang-ylang is tenacious – you will still be able to detect its scent long after opening the bottle.

Ylang-ylang blends well with everything. You can freshen it with citrus and green notes, add a spicy twist with the more pungent orientals, layer it with other florals and enhance it with sweet orientals.

CHAPTER 6

Structuring and Building Your Perfume Blend

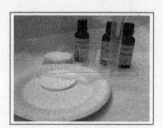

Building a perfume is an enjoyable challenge. You should always experiment by building your perfume blend in small quantities so that there is less wastage should the blend not turn out as expected.

Your blending medium should be inexpensive and disposable, or something that can easily be washed up and reused. Consider using either cotton-wool pads (my preferred method) or washable beakers.

Blending methods
Blending your oils can be carried out in a number of ways.

Blending on cotton-wool pads
The simplest and most effective method is to use the cotton-wool pads: it's quick, easy and relatively inexpensive. Cotton-wool pads allow oils to blend slowly into one another, giving you a first-hand account of the perfume as it develops. You only need a drop or two from a selection oils in order to create a blend.

Blending in beakers
If you don't have cotton-wool pads, drops of oil can be placed into a small plastic or glass beaker, but the beaker will need to be swirled around gently to enable the oils to mix. You'll need several drops of each oil so that there is sufficient to mix together without sticking to the bottom of the beaker. While this method still allows you to enjoy the aroma as it develops, it does work out as slightly more expensive because you need more drops of oil to obtain the same result. If choosing

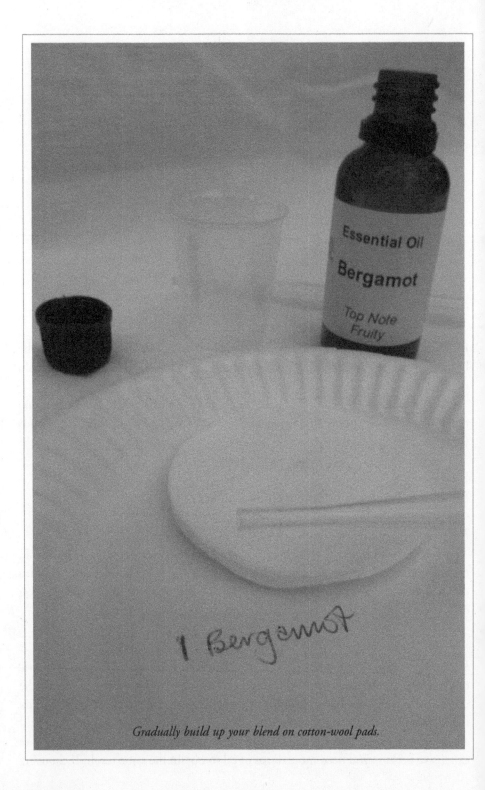

Gradually build up your blend on cotton-wool pads.

the beaker method, follow the exercises described on the following pages, but add the oil drops to the beaker, rather than onto a cotton-wool pad.

Beakers can be washed thoroughly and reused, as opposed to cotton-wool pads, which cannot; however, the latter do make great drawer, trainer or wardrobe scenters. You can also put them in your shoes or boots – but don't forget to remove the pads when you want to wear them!

Creating a simple blend

For this exercise you'll need at least two cotton-wool pads, a plate (preferably a paper plate) and a selection of oils. You will also need pipettes (one per oil) if your oil bottles don't have dripper inserts. You will build two simple blends using similar oils. The only difference will be the base notes.

Step One

Choose the oils for your blend. Start by choosing one from each of the top- and middle-note categories and two from the base-note category. For this exercise I have chosen:

- Bergamot (top note)
- Cucumber (middle note)
- Patchouli (base note)
- Oakmoss (base note)

Step Two

Place 2 cotton-wool pads on the paper plate. Carefully place 1 drop of your top note on each pad. Write your formula directly onto the paper plate. Write the name of the oil and the quantity of drops you have used on each pad. Use a biro so that the ink won't run should it get any oil on it.

Your formula should read:

Cotton-wool pad 1 (Formula 1)	Cotton-wool pad 2 (Formula 2)
1 drop Bergamot	1 drop Bergamot

Step Three

Carefully place a drop of your middle note on each pad. Try to put the middle-note droplet on top of the top note so that the oils have a chance to blend. On the paper plate write the name of the middle-note oil and the quantity of drops you have used on each of the pads. If you accidentally add 2 drops of your middle note, make sure this is recorded.

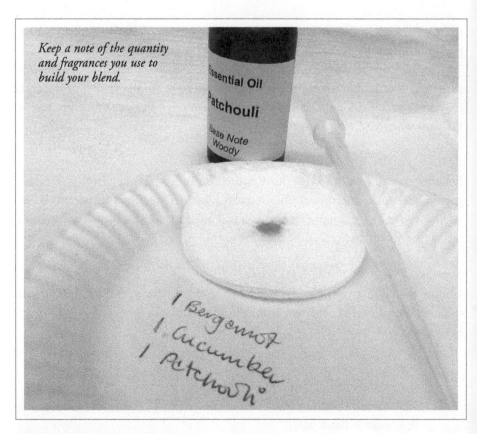

Keep a note of the quantity and fragrances you use to build your blend.

Your formula should now read:

Cotton-wool pad 1 (Formula 1)	Cotton-wool pad 2 (Formula 2)
1 drop Bergamot	1 drop Bergamot
1 drop Cucumber	1 drop Cucumber

Step Four

Pick up one of the pieces of cotton wool and gently waft it under your nose. This allows the oil blend to mingle and lets you experience the two smells as a unit. Place the cotton wool back on the plate read for the base note. At this stage both cotton-wool pads will smell the same because the oils you have used are identical.

Step Five

On 1 of the cotton-wool pads, add 1 drop of the first base note. Write what you have added on the paper plate. On the second pad, add 1 drop of the other base note. Record the oils you've added to your formula on the paper plate. Your paper plate should now contain 2 slightly different formulas.

Your formula should read:

Cotton-wool pad 1 (Formula 1)	Cotton-wool pad 2 (Formula 2)
1 drop Bergamot	1 drop Bergamot
1 drop Cucumber	1 drop Cucumber
1 drop Patchouli	1 drop Oakmoss

Wait a couple of minutes to allow the oils to blend. Pick up the first pad, waft it under your nose and inhale the aroma. Now repeat the exercise with the second pad. You should detect a different aroma.

Pick up cotton-wool pad 1 again and smell it. How does it differ from the second pad? Which aroma do you like best?

The aroma from each cotton-wool pad will continue to mature as the oils settle. Smell them again in 10 minutes to see how they've changed. You can place the pads in small lidded glass jars to allow the blended oils to mature without too much of the aroma escaping. Make sure you label the jars, though, so that you know which concoction it contains.

Step Six
Give your oils a chance to settle. This can easily take an hour or so, due to the slow evaporation of the base notes. Once you feel the smell is no longer changing, the aroma will have developed and the blend is complete.

Record the formula of the blend you wish to use – or record both if you've been lucky enough to create 2 good aromas. Use the blend formulation sheets to keep organised records of your formulation.

Creating a slightly more complex blend
This time you're going to use five different oils. To keep things simple, instead of using 2 cotton-wool pads, you're going to use just 1.

Step One
Choose the oils for your blend. This time choose 2 top-note oils, 2 middle-note oils and 1 base-note oil. For this example I have chosen:

- Bergamot (top note)
- Neroli (top note)
- Rose (middle note)
- Pink Pepper (middle note)
- Vanilla (base note)

Step Two

Carefully place 1 drop of each of the chosen top note oils onto the cotton-wool pad. Try to make sure that the oils are dropped on top of each other, giving them the chance to mingle.

Don't forget to write your formula on the plate or directly onto a formulation sheet. Remember, too, to pick up and waft the cotton wool each time you add a new oil so that you can check how your perfume blend is developing.

Your third formula should read:

Formula 3
1 drop Bergamot
1 drop Neroli

Step Three

Repeat step 2 using the middle notes. Carefully place a drop of each of the middle notes on top of the 2 top notes on the cotton-wool pad. Update your formulation notes so reflect the 2 middle-note additions. Waft the pad under your nose to see how the perfume is developing.

Your formula should now read:

Formula 3
1 drop Bergamot
1 drop Neroli
1 drop Rose
1 drop Pink Pepper

Step Four

Now add the base note and make a record of what you have added. Check how this perfume is developing.

Your final formula should read:

Formula 3
1 drop Bergamot
1 drop Neroli
1 drop Rose
1 drop Pink Pepper
1 drop Vanilla

Leave the cotton-wool pad to mature fully. If you have a spare jar – a clean jam jar with a lid will do nicely – place the pad in the jar and replace the lid. Test the aroma again at 20-minute intervals until the perfume blend has settled. If you're building your blend using the beaker method, put a small piece of cardboard over the beaker to act as a lid. It helps to keep the evaporation to a minimum during this stage.

Creating a structured blend

We are going to repeat the same exercise but this time we are going to structure our perfume slightly differently. You will be using the same five oils you used in the previous exercise, but you will be using a greater quantity of both the bergamot and the rose.

Step One

Line up the oils ready for use. In the example I have kept the same oils as before:

- Bergamot (top note)
- Neroli (top note)
- Rose (middle note)
- Pink Pepper (middle note)
- Vanilla (base note)

Step Two

Carefully place 1 drop of neroli on the cotton-wool pad. This time, instead of 1 drop of bergamot, add 2 drops. Try to make sure that the oils are dropped on top of each other to give them the chance to mingle.

Write your formula on the plate or directly onto a formulation sheet and smell the blend by wafting the pad under your nose. The fourth formula should read:

Formula 4
1 drop Neroli
2 drops Bergamot

Step Three

Add your middle notes as before, but this time add 3 drops of rose. The formula should now read:

Formula 4
1 drop Neroli
2 drops Bergamot
3 drops Rose
1 drop Pink Pepper

Step Four

Now add the base note and make a record of what you have added. Check how this perfume is developing. The final formula should read:

> Formula 4
> 1 drop Neroli
> 2 drops Bergamot
> 3 drops Rose
> 1 drop Pink Pepper
> 1 drop Vanilla

Leave the cotton-wool pad to mature fully; this can be done in a lidded jar or by leaving it on the paper plate. Compare it with the blend that contains the same oils, but less bergamot and rose.

Can you detect the difference? Which aroma do you like best?

Creating a more complex, structured blend

In this exercise you structure and balance your perfume. You will be using a selection of top, middle and base notes but in differing quantities. Choose the oils for your blend. This time choose 2 top-note oils, 3 middle-note oils and 2 base-note oils.

In this exercise the fifth and final blend contains:

> Formula 5
> 2 drops Mandarin (top note)
> 1 drop Petitgrain (top note)
> 2 drops Juniper Berry (middle note)
> 1 drop Lavender (middle note)
> 1 drop Bay (middle note)
> 1 drop Patchouli (base note)
> 3 drops Benzoin (base note)

Build your perfume blend on the cotton-wool pad as per the previous exercises. Leave the pad to mature fully.

The blend you have developed here is more complex than the previous blends. Not only have you used an uneven quantity of top, middle and base notes to give your perfume balance, but you have also used a variety of fragrance families.

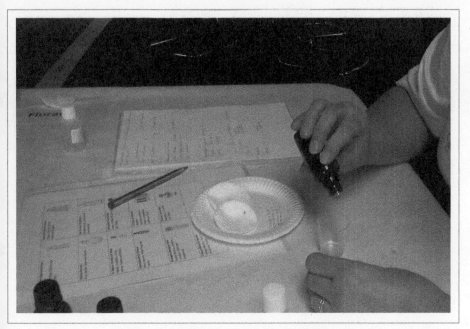

Your perfume blend will need diluting before use.

If we analyse the perfume, we can see that the blend is structured as follows:

Top notes
2 drops Mandarin
1 drop Petitgrain
Total = 3 drops

Middle notes
2 drops Juniper Berry
1 drop Lavender
1 drop Bay
Total = 4 drops

Base notes
1 drop Patchouli
3 drops Benzoin
Total = 4 drops

So our perfume has more base and middle notes than top notes. There is a sufficient volume of top notes to ensure that this perfume has a lively introduction, but it then emerges into a mellowing herbaceous middle layer followed by a lingering woody finish with a slightly sweet twist.

In terms of fragrance family, this blend is broken down as follows:

Fruity fragrance
2 drops Mandarin
1 drop Petitgrain (crossing over into the woody category)
Total = 3 drops

Floral fragrance
1 drop Lavender (crossing over into the fresh and green category)
Total = 1 drop

Fresh and green fragrance
2 drops Juniper Berry
1 drop Bay
Total = 3 drops

Woody fragrance
1 drop Patchouli
Total = 1 drop

Oriental fragrance
3 drops Benzoin
Total = 3 drops

This perfume blend is more adventurous than the blends in the previous exercises. It has layers and depth, and the aroma will change as you experience it.

TO CONCLUDE...

- Build and test your blend using a medium that is inexpensive such as cotton-wool pads. This means you can build your blend using very small amounts of perfume oil. Mistakes can be disposed of without too much expense!
- Build similar blends on cotton-wool pads, changing the blend as you wish. The pads can be placed in a small lidded jar to allow them to continue to develop over a number of hours.

HOW TO CREATE A LARGER VOLUME
OF PERFUME BLEND

Once you've mastered the art of creating a blend using cotton-wool pads you can move onto the next step, which is to create the same blend but in sufficient quantities to use as a base for your perfume or other scented product.

The first stage involves a little maths because you will need to scale up your cotton-wool perfume blend to make enough volume for your scented product. The calculation is easy once you get the hang of it, but it may appear a little challenging at first.

Measuring in parts, not drops

Perfume oil formulas are usually referred to as 'parts' rather than 'drops'. This allows us to understand the proportion of the oils used regardless of the actual quantity.

Using the blends made in the previous exercise, if we refer to Formula 1 in drops, then it only enables us to make 3 drops of the blend. If we refer to it in parts, this allows us to make any quantity we like as long as we stick to the equal proportion of perfume oils.

From now on we will refer to our perfume blend in parts rather than drops.

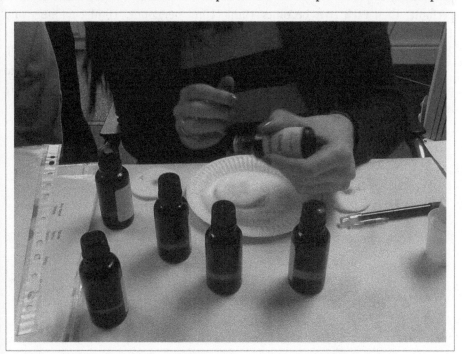

Creating a blend of oils on a cotton-wool pad.

If your perfume blend contains 1 drop of 3 different oils, then it's easy to convert from drops to parts. All you need to do is look for the lowest part number (which is 1) and divide all the other parts by this number. The maths is easy here; any number divided by 1 remains the same. Therefore Formula 1 is easily converted into parts.

Formula 1 contains:
1 drop Bergamot
1 drop Cucumber
1 drop Patchouli

The maths formula is $1 \div 1 = 1$, therefore we simply substitute the word 'part' for 'drop'. So formula 1 is now written as:

Formula 1
1 part Bergamot
1 part Cucumber
1 part Patchouli

Using this principal, no matter how much of the perfume blend you make, the proportion, or parts, will always be the same. For example, if you make 30ml of perfume, then each part becomes 10ml (10ml bergamot, 10ml cucumber and 10ml patchouli). If you make 600ml of the perfume blend, then each part becomes 200ml, so you would use 200ml bergamot, 200ml cucumber and 200ml patchouli.

Formulas 2 and 3 (from the previous exercise) are also easy to translate into parts as they, too, have an equal number of drops of each perfume oil. Formula 2 is now correctly written as:

Formula 2
1 part Bergamot
1 part Cucumber
1 part Oakmoss

Formula 3 is now correctly written as:

Formula 3
1 part Bergamot
1 part Neroli
1 part Rose
1 part Pink Pepper
1 part Vanilla

Using a mathematical formula to convert drops into parts

Let's look at converting drops into parts for formulas where the number of drops is not equal. We'll start by converting the following formula into parts:

2 drops Neroli
2 drops Bergamot
4 drops Lily of the Valley
2 drops Violet
4 drops Benzoin

First, check your formula to find the perfume oil with the lowest number of drops. In our example, neroli, bergamot and violet have only 2 drops whereas lily of the valley and benzoin have 4. Therefore our lowest number is 2.

The final part of the calculation is to divide the number of drops for each perfume oil by the lowest number (in this case, 2) to get the number of parts. It's easier than it sounds— truly! Our calculations are therefore carried out as follows:

Neroli – 2 drops $2 \div 2 = 1$
Bergamot – 2 drops $2 \div 2 = 1$
Lily of the Valley – 4 drops $4 \div 2 = 2$
Violet – 2 drops $2 \div 2 = 1$
Benzoin – 4 drops $4 \div 2 = 2$

Therefore our formula should be written as:

1 part Neroli
1 part Bergamot
2 parts Lily of the Valley
1 part Violet
2 parts Benzoin

Let's perform that calculation again using the following perfume formula:

3 drops Lemon
12 drops Orange
6 drops Bergamot
6 drops Lavender
3 drops Rosemary
3 drops Coriander
3 drops Patchouli
9 drops Oakmoss

Our perfume formula is looking a little more complex, but the mathematical calculation remains the same. First, check the formula for the lowest measurement. In this case, it's 3, since patchouli, rosemary and lemon are included at only 3 drops each.

Next, divide the number of drops for each oil by three. This will result in the perfume formula being correctly displayed as:

1 part Lemon (3 ÷3 = 1)
4 parts Orange (12 ÷3 = 4)
2 parts Bergamot (6 ÷3 = 2)
2 parts Lavender (6 ÷3 = 2)
1 part Rosemary (3 ÷3 = 1)
1 part Coriander (3 ÷3 = 1)
1 part Patchouli (3 ÷3 = 1)
3 parts Oakmoss (9 ÷3 = 3)

There! It's easy once you know what you're doing!

What to do when the maths won't work

Of course, there are occasions where the number of drops can't be divided evenly by the smallest quantity.

An example of this occurs in the following formula:

6 drops Petitgrain
5 drops Grapefruit
5 drops Geranium
3 drops Bay
3 drops Cedar
4 drops Sandalwood
2 drops Vetiver

Following the normal calculation rules, you can see that 2 is the smallest number. However, you cannot divide 5 (the number of grapefruit and geranium drops) or 3 (the number of bay and cedar drops) by 2.

The good news is that this means you don't have to do any mathematics at all – simply leave the numbers as they are but refer to them as parts rather than drops.

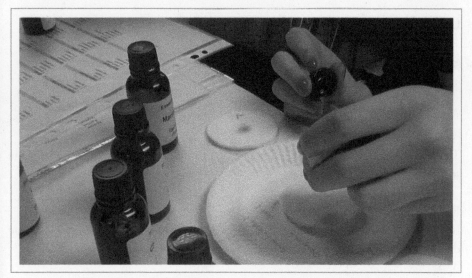

Keep a note of each oil, plus the quantity you use in your blend.

Therefore the perfume formula will be written as:

6 parts Petitgrain
5 parts Grapefruit
5 parts Geranium
3 parts Bay
3 parts Cedar
4 parts Sandalwood
2 parts Vetiver

Converting perfume oil from weight into parts

While we've been using drops as our perfume oil measurement, there may be times when you will work with the weight of perfume oil rather than the number of drops.

The maths formula you've already mastered is exactly the same for converting the weights into parts.

Example 1
In this example our perfume formula is:

10g Lavender
5g Patchouli
20g Lemon
10g Geranium

Using the same calculation discussed earlier, the blend should be referred to as:

> 2 parts Lavender
> 1 part Patchouli
> 4 parts Lemon
> 2 parts Geranium

To calculate the parts, I've divided each of perfume oil by 5, since patchouli is the smallest quantity, weighing only 5g.

Example 2
In this example, the lowest weight is 2g, meaning that all other weights should be divided by 2. Let's take a perfume that has the following ingredients as its blend:

> 18g Bergamot
> 6g Orange
> 5g Mandarin
> 2g Lemon Grass
> 2g Rosewood

Since you can't divide 5 (mandarin 5g) by 2, leave the measurements as they are, but refer to them as parts rather than as grams. The blend for Example 2 should be referred to as:

> 18 parts Bergamot
> 6 parts Orange
> 5 parts Mandarin
> 2 parts Lemon Grass
> 2 parts Rosewood

TO CONCLUDE...

- By referring to your perfume blend in parts, you make your perfume scalable, i.e. each part may be calculated to weigh 1g, 10g or even 100g, depending on how much perfume you want to make. It is rather like working in percentages, only we refer to the perfume measurement as parts.

PUTTING TOGETHER YOUR PERFUME BLEND

Once you've created your perfume blend using the cotton-wool pad method, your blend needs to be made into a perfume oil, which can then be diluted to make it suitable for use on skin.

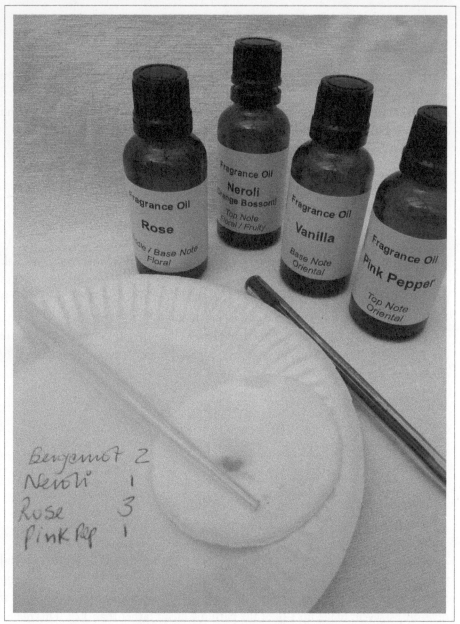

Use a selection of different perfume notes to create a structured, memorable blend.

Start with a simple blend, such as the simple example used on page 73, then move onto more complex blends.

Example 1 contains:
1 part Bergamot
1 part Cucumber
1 part Patchouli

If you wish to make 12g of perfume blend (before dilution), another calculation is called for. The formula for converting our perfume blend from parts to actual measurements is done by adding up the number of parts (in this case 3), and dividing it into our required amount (in this case 12g).

number of parts
↓
Our calculation is 12 ÷ 3 = 4 ◄— new value for each part
↑
total amount required

Each part needs to be multiplied by four to make 12g of perfume blend in total.

If each part is multiplied by 4, each part becomes 4g. This means you need to mix 4g bergamot with 4g cucumber and 4g patchouli. You can see that the total is 12g so you know you've done the correct calculations.

Repeat that exercise on a few other perfume blends just to make sure you're comfortable with the calculation required. For each example you want to make 12g of perfume blend.

Example 2
1 part Neroli
1 part Bergamot
2 parts Lily of the Valley
1 part Violet
2 parts Benzoin
Total = 7 parts

As you can probably already work out, 12 (12g, the weight of the perfume blend you want to make) is not easily divisible by seven. In this case we always make up more perfume blend than we need to keep the calculations simple. Since 14 *is* divisible by seven, make up 14g of the perfume blend rather than 12g. This makes the calculations work out as follows:

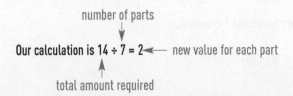

number of parts

Our calculation is 14 ÷ 7 = 2 ◄— new value for each part

total amount required

Each individual part becomes 2g, so the perfume blend will need to be measured out as follows:

2g Neroli
2g Bergamot
4g Lily of the Valley
2g Violet
4g Benzoin
Total = 14g

You now have enough for 12g of perfume blend with 2g left over.

Always round up the total required to make your maths easy. Trying to calculate using decimal points and trying to weigh fractions of a gram isn't easy, so just round the required weight of your perfume up to a number that can be divided by the number of parts. You'll have some perfume blend left over, but you will have saved yourself a mathematical headache!

Example 3
1 part Grapefruit
3 parts Orange
2 parts Bergamot
2 parts Basil
1 part Rosemary
1 part Coriander
2 part Patchouli
Total = 12 parts

This calculation is refreshingly simple. Each part becomes 1g.

number of parts

Our calculation is 12 ÷ 12 = 1 ◄— new value for each part

total amount required

Therefore the blend becomes:

1g Grapefruit
3g Orange
2g Bergamot
2g Basil
1g Rosemary
1g Coriander
2g Patchouli

Example 4

This time I'm changing the formula slightly. Instead of 12g final perfume blend, I need 50g. The maths calculation is exactly the same, but using 50 as the number to divide the number of parts with instead of 12.

6 parts Petitgrain
5 parts Lemon
5 parts Galbanum
5 parts Lavender
2 parts Salty Sea Dog
1 part Cedar
1 part Honey
Total = 25 parts

number of parts
↓
Our calculation is 50 ÷ 25 = 2 ◄— new value for each part
↑
total amount required

This perfume blend needs to be made up of:

12g Petitgrain
10g Lemon
10g Galbanum
10g Lavender
4g Salty Sea Dog
2g Cedar
2g Honey

TO CONCLUDE...

- In order to scale up perfume into larger quantities, you must perform a calculation. This calculation requires you to know the total amount of perfume blend you want to make. Divide the total amount required by the number of parts in your perfume blend and you will know the weight required for each part.

- Multiply the number of parts in your blend by the calculated weight to determine the total amount required.

- Work out how to convert your perfume blend into drops, parts, ml and/or grams. Accurate calculations and recording will help you enormously if you wish to repeat a successful perfume blend to make it again (and again!).

- Once you've mastered the art of using the calculation formula, the maths gets easier.

CHAPTER 7

How to Dilute Your Perfume Blends

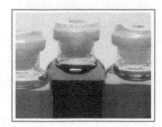

As stated earlier, the perfume blends you create are too strong to go straight onto your body or clothing and must be diluted before they can be used. There are many liquids you can use to dilute perfume oils. These are referred to as dilutants, diluents or solvents. The dilutant you choose depends on the final product you're making and your personal preference.

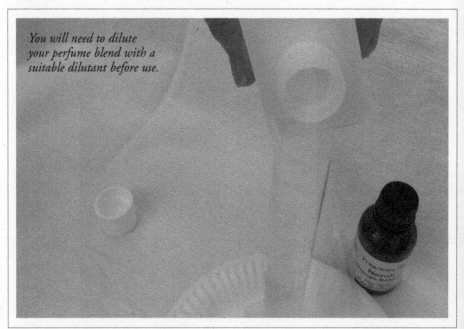

You will need to dilute your perfume blend with a suitable dilutant before use.

CHOOSING A SUITABLE DILUTANT

Many diluting ingredients are used in perfume-creation. Their role is to dilute perfume oils to make them safe to go on skin, whether as a perfume or perfumed oil.

Water

While many commercial perfumes may use water mixed with solvents to dilute their perfume, I avoid the use of water because it can be a breeding ground for bacteria unless you include a preservative. There are plenty of other ingredients that make equally good, if not better, dilutants and also avoid the need for a preservative. I recommend the use of these so that you can avoid the water/preservative issue altogether.

In addition, your perfume oils won't blend into water because the two ingredients, oil and water, don't bind together naturally. If you simply place perfume oils in water you will see little blobs of perfume oil floating around. Shaking the container will disperse the oil, but only for a short time.

Carrier oil

Your perfume oil blend can be mixed with carrier oils such as jojoba oil, sweet almond oil and coconut oil. Perfume oils will distribute evenly in carrier oil, but they will create an initial oily residue on your skin. If your clothing rubs against the oil it may transfer and cause a permanent mark.

Perfumers' alcohol

Perfumers' alcohol is usually a blend of dilutants, each chosen for their ability to slow the evaporation of perfume oil as well as for their super-soft feel on the skin. My preferred perfumers' alcohol is a blend of denatured alcohol, isopropyl myristate and dipropylene glycol. This has been specially formulated to slow the evaporation of the perfume while having a lovely silky glide on skin.

Denatured alcohol

Ethanol or ethyl alcohol makes an excellent perfume dilutant. Alcohol mixes with oils, ensuring that the perfume blend is distributed evenly, but more importantly it will evaporate, allowing your perfume to waft into the air.

To denature alcohol, a little hexane – or similarly revolting-tasting ingredient – is added to ensure that it is too disgusting to drink, and is therefore exempt from regular duty on alcohol. Denatured alcohol is listed as 'alcohol denat' on perfume-label ingredients listings.

Vodka

Yes, you can use vodka! In fact, any alcohol will do, but vodka is the best because it is pretty much odourless and clear. Cheap and cheerful, rough and ready is fine, but I do recommend high-grade, 100%-proof vodka if you can stretch to it.

However, if you plan to start a business making and selling perfumes, you should consider using perfumers' alcohol or alcohol denat, as you won't be able to sell perfume made with vodka or other alcohol that requires additional duty to be paid on it.

Isopropyl myristate

Isopropyl myristate, or IPM, is a clear, non-alcohol-based dilutant that holds aromas well. It is derived from the myristic fatty acid found in oils such as coconut oil. It has an initial mildly greasy feel, but this is soon absorbed by the skin.

Silicone

Most silicone liquids are non-greasy and evaporate slowly, making them an ideal base for diluting perfume oils. Look for cyclomethicone, dimethicone or cyclopentasiloxane; these can be used in both roll-on perfumes and sprays.

Dipropylene glycol

Dipropylene glycol, or DPG, is a colourless, odourless liquid that enables your perfume-oil blends to mix with water. While this allows you to dilute your perfume with water, making it go further, it will still require the addition of a preservative to prevent any mould or bacteria growth. DPG does not need to be used with water and can be also mixed with alcohol denat or perfumers' alcohol to thin it down a little. DPG is excellent at slowing the speed of evaporation and is skin-safe.

Floral waters

Floral waters are a by-product of essential oil steam distillation: the water left behind after the essential oil has been taken off. The waters themselves hold the aroma of the original plant material and can be used on their own or to enhance a perfume. Rose floral water is an excellent way of including a natural aroma of oil without having to use the expensive essential oil.

However, floral waters are not immune to the growth of bacteria and mould so still require the addition of a preservative if they are to be combined with your perfume oil. As with regular water, the use of a dispersant such as DPG is required to allow the perfume blend to disperse in water without leaving oil droplets floating on the surface.

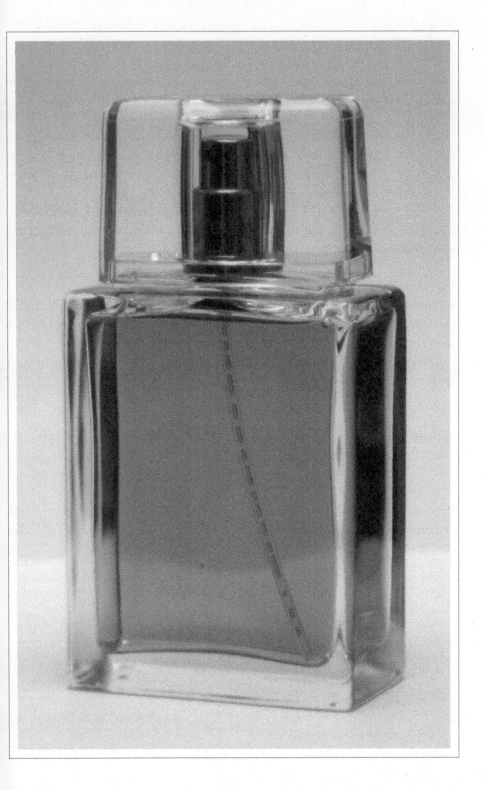

OTHER DILUTANTS USED IN PERFUMED PRODUCTS

Many other ingredients make suitable perfume oil dilutants. Each has a different function and needs to be chosen according to the product you're making.

Sulphonated castor oil
Sulphonated castor oil (also known as Turkey Red Oil) is a solubizer used for dispersing oils in water. You can use it with floral waters, purified (deionised/distilled) waters, spring water and tap water.

Sulphonated castor oil is not usually used as a base for perfumes, but makes an ideal base for bath oils and ensures that the bathwater becomes moisturising and scented without droplets of oils floating on the surface.

Polysorbates
Polysorbates also allow perfume blends to dissolve in water. Polysorbate 80, derived from olive oil, is suitable for bath oils because you can blend it with other oils such as jojoba, sweet almond or avocado as well as your perfume blend.

Polysorbate 20, derived from coconut oil, is suitable for a room spray or body spray because it's lighter, reducing the chances of an oily spray.

Sucragel
Sucragel is similar to the polysorbates and can be used with oils and water as a room spray and a bath oil.

Ressassol
Ressassol is a branded product used in room and linen sprays. It mixes well with perfume oils and all water types and allows the blend to remain clear rather than cloudy.

TO CONCLUDE...
- Dilute your perfume oil before you use it and in order to make it safe to go on your skin.
- Many different solutions can be used to dilute perfume oils. The dilutant you choose is either determined by the style of your final perfumed product or simply by personal preference.

DILUTING YOUR PERFUME OIL BLEND

Diluting a perfume oil blend is as simple as making up a drink of orange squash using orange cordial and water. The method is similar to making orange squash but you use your perfume blend instead of orange cordial and your chosen dilutant instead of water.

When making orange squash you put in as much water as necessary for your personal taste. Use only a little water and the squash will possibly be too strong and sweet. Use too much, and the drink may be watery and not as flavoursome as you might like.

Similarly, when diluting a perfume blend, the volume of dilutant you use will determine the style of the final perfumed product.

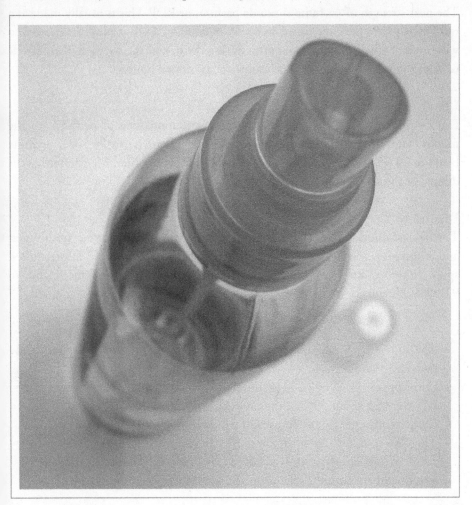

Understanding perfume strengths

There are varying strengths of perfume available. Each is made from the same blend of perfume oil, but thinned with different strengths of dilutant.

Parfum

The strongest type of perfume is pure perfume (*parfum*) which understandably is also the most expensive form. Pure perfume is usually sold in small bottles and applied to wrists or neck by dabbing the perfume directly onto the skin rather than spraying. The ratio of perfume to dilutant is usually up to 30% perfume blend to 70% perfumers' alcohol or other dilutant.

Eau de parfum

The next strength of perfume is eau de parfum, or EDP. This is usually made at a ratio of 10–15% perfume blend to 85–90% dilutant. EDP is ideal for those who wish to apply their perfume only once during the day, as the strength of an eau de parfum should allow the perfume aroma to last several hours.

Eau de toilette & aftershave

Eau de toilette (EDT) is probably the most common style of perfume on the market. The ratio of perfume to dilutant in eau de toilette is usually 5–8% perfume blend to 92-95% dilutant. This is usually sold in spray bottles. Men's aftershave is diluted at the same ratio as eau de toilette.

Eau fraîche/body spray

The lightest dilution of perfume is eau fraîche, which literally means 'fresh water' and is also known simply as body spray. These are usually packaged in pressurised spray canisters and are diluted at a strength of 1–3% perfume blend to 97-99% dilutants.

TO CONCLUDE...

- The amount of dilutant you use will determine the style of your final perfume product.
- The strongest-smelling of all perfume products is parfum, where the perfume oils make up about 30% of the product.
- The next-strongest is eau de parfum which contains 10–15% perfume blend. Then we have eau de toilette and aftershaves, where between 5–8% of the final product is the perfume blend. Finally, eau fraîche, which is the weakest-smelling of all as only 1–3% of the final product is perfume oil blend.

DILUTING DIFFERENT-STRENGTH PERFUME PRODUCTS

Once you've created your perfume blend you need to dilute it to make it safe to use as a perfumed product. The more dilutant you use, the weaker your perfume will be, although even the weakest perfume, eau fraîche, will still hold its smell for an hour or so, depending on the formula.

How to calculate the volume of dilutant required

The chart below shows how to calculate the amount of dilutant you will need to use to create your finished perfumed product. Although the example shows the calculation for 2g of perfume blend, you can use the calculation column to work out how much dilutant you need for any quantity of your blend.

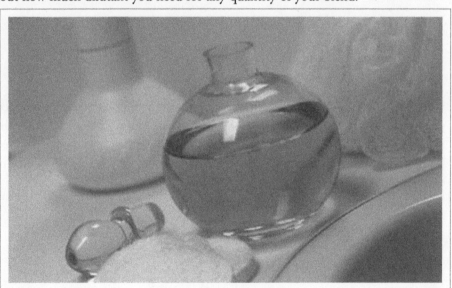

Dilution chart

Perfume Type	Quantity of Blend	Quantity of Perfume Required	Calculation Dilutant	% Ratio (perfume blend to dilutant)
Parfum	2g	8g	Perfume blend x 4	20 : 80 %
Eau de parfum	2g	18g	Perfume blend x 9	10 : 90 %
EDT / aftershave	2g	38g	Perfume blend x 19	5 : 95 %
Eau fraîche	2g	98g	Perfume blend x 49	2 : 98%

Diluting your perfume blend using different strengths

In this example we will work out how to dilute my *Italian Garden* perfume blend to make a perfume, an eau de parfum, an eau de toilette or aftershave and an eau fraîche. The *Italian Garden* perfume blend is structured as follows:

8 parts Bergamot
8 parts Mandarin
7 parts Neroli
2 parts Fig
3 parts Lilac
6 parts Plum
8 parts Rose
4 parts Benzoin
3 parts Honey
1 part Clove
Total = 50 parts

Since you'll be diluting 5ml of perfume oil to make the finished perfume product, you must first convert the parts into physical measurements to make up 5ml. The formula for this is listed on page 88, but to recap: divide the total amount required (5ml) by the number of parts (50) in order to determine the weight or volume of each individual part.

number of parts

Our calculation is 5 ÷ 50 = 0.1 ◄—— new value for each part

total amount required

Using this formula you can see that each of part is equal to 0.1ml. You now need to multiply each part in the formula above by 0.1 in order to calculate how much of each oil is needed.

The calculations and results:

Formula in parts	Calculation required to convert to ml	Calculation required to convert to drops
	parts x 0.1 = x ml	30 x no. ml = no. drops
8 parts Bergamot	8 x 0.1 = 0.8ml	30 x 0.8 = 24 drops
8 parts Mandarin	8 x 0.1 = 0.8ml	30 x 0.8 = 24 drops
7 parts Neroli	7 x 0.1 = 0.7ml	30 x 0.7 = 21 drops
2 parts Fig	2 x 0.1 = 0.2ml	30 x 0.2 = 6 drops
3 parts Lilac	3 x 0.1 = 0.3ml	30 x 0.3 = 9 drops
6 parts Plum	6 x 0.1 = 0.6ml	30 x 0.6 = 18 drops
8 parts Rose	8 x 0.1 = 0.8ml	30 x 0.8 = 24 drops
4 parts Benzoin	4 x 0.1 = 0.4ml	30 x 0.4 = 12 drops
3 parts Honey	3 x 0.1 = 0.3ml	30 x 0.3 = 9 drops
1 part Clove	1 x 0.1 = 0.1ml	30 x 0.1 = 3 drops
Total = 50 parts	Total = 5ml	Total = 150 drops

If you don't have an accurate method of measuring such small quantities, you may need to measure in drops. Allowing for 30 drops per gram, the last column has worked out the number of drops you need for each perfume oil.

Counting drops in large volumes requires complete concentration; a slight distraction and you could lose count. Weighing, or using an accurate volume measuring device such as a measuring cylinder, is much more reliable. If you do dispense drop by drop and find your calculations require half a drop, round down rather than up.

Our 5ml perfume oil can now be made up using either the amounts in column two or the number of drops in column 3. Whichever method you use, you should end up with approximately 5ml of the perfume blend.

Calculating the dilutant required to blend your perfume oil

The next and final stage before bottling your perfume is to dilute it. The chart below shows you how much perfume dilutant you will need to dilute a 5ml perfume blend into a parfum, an eau de parfum, an eau de toilette/aftershave or an eau fraîche.

It is similar to the previous chart, but uses 5ml perfume blend instead of 2ml/grams. The last column shows you the total quantity you would make rather than the ratio used. The total quantity is the amount of perfume oil (5ml) added to the quantity of dilutant, which differs according to the final perfume product you wish to make.

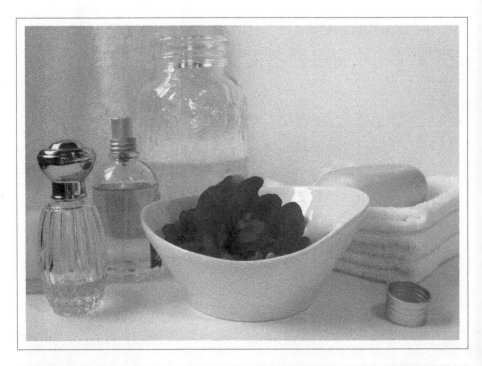

Perfume type	Quantity of perfume blend	Quantity of dilutant required	Calculation	Total quantity made from 5ml perfume blend
Parfum	5ml	20ml	Perfume blend x 4	25ml parfum
Eau de parfum	5ml	45ml	Perfume blend x 9	5ml EDP
EDT / aftershave	5ml	95ml	Perfume blend x 19	100ml EDT /aftershave
Eau fraîche	5ml	245ml	Perfume blend x 49	250ml eau fraîche

TO CONCLUDE...

- The amount of dilution ingredient you need is calculated according to the style of the perfume product you want to make and how much you want to make.
- Once you've decided what strength of dilution you require, work out how much dilutant to use. This can be calculated easily by multiplying the volume of perfume oils as follows:

    Parfum – multiply perfume oil weight by 4
    EDP – multiply perfume oil weight by 9
    EDT – multiply perfume oil weight by 19
    Eau fraîche – multiply perfume oil weight by 49

Mixing the dilutant and perfume oil

Using the chart on the previous page, you can now create an eau de toilette or aftershave version of the *Italian Garden* blend. Because you already know what is going into the blend, there's no need to test it on cotton-wool pads. Instead, simply place the oils directly into a measuring beaker or measuring cylinder.

Line up the oils that you need for the Italian Garden blend and add the required volume, either by measuring or counting drops, into the beaker or cylinder. It doesn't matter in which order you add the oils. You can add the top notes first, then the middle, moving down to the base notes, or you can start at the base notes and work up. Even if you add some middle notes, then top notes, then base notes, then another middle note followed by another top note, it doesn't matter. By the time the oils in your perfume blend have mingled, merged and settled, the perfume will smell the same, regardless of the order in which the oils were added.

Once the perfume blend has been completed, add 95ml your chosen dilutant and give the mixture a stir. If your beaker or cylinder isn't big enough to hold 95ml, add what you can fit in, pour this strong dilution into your perfume bottle then add more of the dilution to the beaker or cylinder. Swirl it around a little in the beaker to pick up any of the strongly diluted perfume oil residue. Pour this into the perfume bottle so that it mixes with the previous pour.

Repeat this process until you have added all 95ml of your dilutant to your perfume blend in the perfume bottle. Put the lid or spray attachment on to the bottle and give it a gentle shake to ensure the perfume oils and dilutant are thoroughly mixed.

Bottling the perfume

While pouring a liquid into a bottle sounds easy in theory, pouring perfume can often be a little tricky – and what a shame if any were to be spilled. A steady hand is an advantage! If your measuring cylinder has a pouring spout and you have a relatively steady hand, then you should have no problem at all, but if you're using a little plastic beaker, there is a chance that the perfume will overshoot the neck of the bottle and dribble down the sides.

One way of overcoming this is to squeeze the rim of the beaker so that it creates a much smaller pouring space. However, if your beaker is made of sturdy plastic, squeezing to this extent may not be possible. If this is the case, use a clean pipette to dispense the perfume from the beaker to the bottle. However, if you are dispensing, say, 100ml of perfume, then dispensing in 5ml portions is not for the impatient!

By far the easiest method is to use a tiny funnel. You need a funnel with a spout that is thin enough to go into the neck of the bottle, and one that's light enough not to make your smaller perfume bottles top-heavy and prone to falling over while pouring.

Whichever method you find easiest, always make sure that you're pouring with one hand and holding the bottle firmly with the other. This eliminates the chances of it falling over while pouring.

Never overfill a bottle – just fill it up to the neck. If your bottle has a spray attachment, then the tubing and mechanism need space and may displace some of your perfume upon insertion, causing it to spill out. If you initially under-fill, you can always top up when you've checked how much space the spray attachment takes up.

TO CONCLUDE...

- Diluting your perfume is the last stage of making your perfume. Once you have decided which dilutant to use and how much you need, the dilution can take place.
- If you don't have a container big enough to dilute your perfume oil, partially dilute it in the container, pour it into the bottle and add the remaining dilution liquid directly into the bottle – or via the container to pick up any perfume oil residue.
- Pouring into the bottle needs a steady hand. Using a funnel will make pouring easier, but be sure your bottle is held steady so that the funnel doesn't make it top-heavy and topple over.

PERFUME-MAKING STAGES CHECKLIST

We've worked through the stages of choosing perfume oils based on your chosen fragrance type and structured your perfume so that it has a good balance and won't disappear too quickly.

You've tested a number of perfume oils by blending them on cotton-wool pads to see how they work together, both initially and once they have had a chance to settle. You've chosen a blend that worked well to make into a perfume and converted the amount of your chosen blend into drops, grams or millilitres (ml).

You considered different diluting ingredients and chosen one you prefer. You then made a decision as to whether to make a parfum, an eau de parfum, an eau de toilette or a light body spray. Your decision required you to do a little maths to work out the amount of perfume blend and dilution solution required. That sorted, you then made up your perfume oil blend and mixed it with the dilution solution.

And finally you poured it into the bottle. That's your first beautiful perfume made. Your perfume-making process is complete! Congratulations!

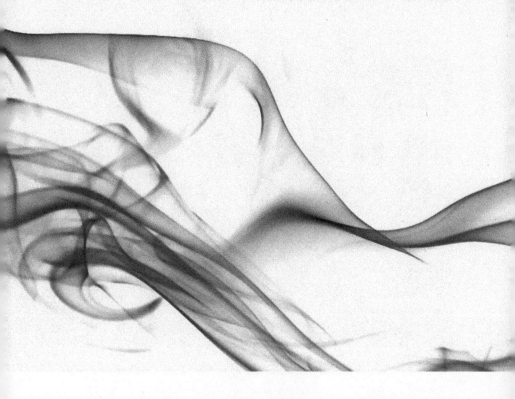

CHAPTER 8

Finishing Touches

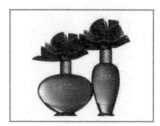

The enjoyment and hard work involved in making a perfume go into its design and structure, but there are many other factors that make a fragrance exciting and/or commercially successful and enjoyable to wear.

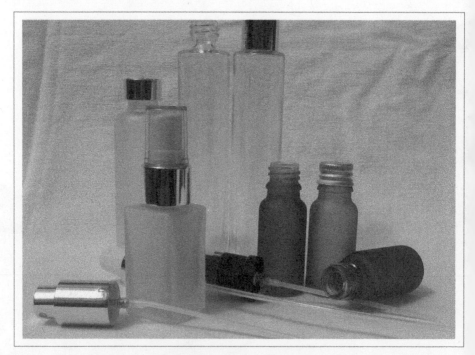

You will need to find a selection of perfume bottles, roll-ons and sprays.

PACKAGING

Research tells us that 75 per cent of customers who go into a shop to buy perfume enter without having already decided which perfume they're going to buy. While part of that decision-making process is determined by the perfume's smell, research also suggests that appealing and attractive packaging is the most important factor. On shop shelves, where there are literally hundreds of perfumes to choose from, bottles that look chic and stylish are more likely to make us want to try a perfume than those perfumes packaged in plain 'boring' bottles.

As a perfume manufacturer you need to consider several options when choosing the right container for your perfume. As well as visual appeal, you also want to ensure that your perfumes are packaged in practical and convenient containers that don't cost you the earth.

Perfume applicators

You can apply perfume in several ways: spraying, dabbing, rolling and rubbing. The method chosen depends on the perfume-bottle applicator.

Perfume dabbers

Dabbing your perfume is perfect for the strongest, most expensive style of all – parfum. Bottles that require you to dab perfume usually come with a large glass stopper that fits snugly into the neck. The bottle needs to be tilted so that some of the perfume touches the stopper, which is then removed and dabbed onto your neck, wrists and anywhere else that you wish to apply the scent.

Perfume put on in this way is applied directly to the skin, not the clothing. Dabbers ensure that every drop of perfume is worn on the skin. There is little or no wastage applying your perfume in this way, but unless the bottle's lid can be secured in some fashion, it is not ideal to carry around in your handbag.

Other perfumes that get dabbed on are the little vials given as free gifts or samplers. The lids of these often snap off, or are unscrewed, revealing a long plastic applicator that you use to apply the perfume.

Roll-on

Perfume roll-on bottles are very practical. There is no chance of spillage, so they're ideal to carry around in your handbag or pocket. The roller ball is clicked into its socket when first closed, sealing the bottle and making it very difficult for the perfume liquid to leak. The perfume can be rolled on directly onto your skin so there is no wastage. Perfume roll-on bottles are suitable for eau de parfum, eau de toilette and lighter fragrances.

Sprays

Possibly the easiest and most popular form of applying perfume comes in the form of a spray. This is definitely the most wasteful of all the applications, as up to half the perfume is lost into the air rather than landing on your skin. It does, however, allow you to spray perfume liberally over your body and clothing and is definitely better suited to eau de toilette and lighter daytime sprays.

Spraying onto clothing can help limit direct contact between skin and perfume. This is a useful if you find your skin is a little sensitive to perfume.

Some spray perfumes, especially the lighter body sprays, come in pressurised canisters. This method of storage helps to reduce contact between the perfume and the air, which in turn can help keep the perfume fresher for longer. See page 113, 'Storing your perfume, for more information on shelf life. It is usually the light, daytime body sprays such as eau fraîche that are sold in pressurised canisters.

Screwtop perfume bottles

If you're fortunate enough to purchase a perfume packaged in a screwtop bottle, you'll be able to reuse the bottle once the perfume is gone. Make sure that you wash the bottle thoroughly in hot soapy water, then rinse it in clean hot water to remove all traces of the perfume – and hopefully the aroma.

Screwtop bottles are not leak-proof, and the contents can be easily accessed. Brand-named perfumes are not usually sold in this style of bottle.

Crimped perfume bottles

Most perfume bottles have their spray top crimped onto the neck of the bottle. This not only prevents the top from coming loose by accident, but it also prevents it coming off at all. Unfortunately, this means that you cannot reuse the bottle once the perfume is finished.

Crimping the spray attachment onto the bottle requires a special tool that squeezes the attachment over a little lip at the top of the perfume bottle neck. As it squeezes it bends the material of the spray attachment so that it grips the lid lip in such a way that it cannot be undone. This process is an excellent method of making sure that the attachment cannot come loose and therefore makes the bottle of perfume spill-proof and leak-proof.

Perfume containers disguised as jewellery

Perfume houses are always looking at new, innovative ways of helping you carry your perfume around with you without having to worry about leakage, breakage or additional heavy items in your handbag. Some perfumes are available in exclusive editions that are packed in items of jewellery, such as amulets, pendant necklaces and rings. While these may be convenient, the perfume container will be small and if it isn't refillable, it will be of limited use time-wise.

Solid perfume containers

Solid perfume can be packed in any suitable container and can easily be small enough to carry in a handbag. Because it is a solid perfume, there is no risk of spillage. However, solid perfume is susceptible to heat, and if allowed to get too warm will soften to the point of melting.

TO CONCLUDE...

- How you apply your perfume depends upon the applicator that is integral to the perfume bottle. Some are leak-proof, some prevent the perfume from being wasted and some are more practical when it comes to carrying the perfume on your person or in your handbag.
- An ideal way of securing the cap fittings is to crimp the fixture onto the bottle neck. This may not be feasible for handmade perfumes, however, since the crimper tool can be costly.
- Screwtop bottles are probably your best solution, although do bear in mind that these cannot guarantee leak-proof bottles since the tops can loosen.

Packaging design

Package design is of prime importance to the success of any product, and even more so for a perfume. Not only do perfume bottles need to look alluring and tempting on shop shelves, but since they will adorn bathroom shelves and dressing tables it is essential that they continue to look attractive and appealing as well as contain the most delectable elixirs.

It may be that you know exactly what perfume you want to purchase since you have succumbed to advertising, enjoyed wearing a sample or been delighted with a perfume worn by someone else. While it's possibly the aroma that initially makes you seek out a perfume, many fragrances are bought as gifts, and it is then that the bottle or container will be as an important attention-grabber as the aroma.

A perfume container should identify with the perfume it holds – but it would seem that in the world of perfume, there are no hard and set rules. Perfumes have been packaged in all sorts of shapes and materials.

Memorable designs

Jean Paul Gaultier puts his perfumes and aftershaves in a beautiful woman's-torso-shaped bottle, then hides the bottle in a tin – concealing the bottle until the tin is opened. Angel by Thierry Mugler is packaged in a star-shaped bottle where one of the points on the star is the spray dispenser. Paloma Picasso was famed for her love of everything red, from lipstick to gloves, dresses and hats. Her signature perfume is poured into a black bottle packaged in a red box.

One of my particular favourites is Lola by Marc Jacobs, where the perfume container is a regular purple oval(ish)-shaped glass bottle but the lid, which is almost the same size as the bottle, is a big, multilayered flower – worthy of perching on any hat at Ascot!

Special shapes and crazy ideas aren't limited just to ladies' perfumes. A bottle of men's Diesel Fuel for Life aftershave is packaged in a bottle covered in hand-sewn leather to give it a more masculine appeal, while a bottle of Giorgio Armani Attitude looks as if it's a cigarette lighter.

Very often the packaging is worth more than the contents inside. A bottle of Shalimar recently went on e-Bay for a starting price of $1,500.00 (approximately £900). The bottle was a limited edition made by Baccarat exclusively for Guerlain.

Lancôme's L'Air du Temps also had limited-edition versions, packaged in bottles made by Lalique. These are still collector's items today and sell for far more than the original price of the product, even though the perfume contents have long gone.

TO CONCLUDE...

- Even though it is the perfume that is the required product, perfume designer houses add extra appeal to perfumes by packaging them in a unique, unusual and eye-catching container, hoping this added charm will make them more likely to sell.

Sourcing your bottles

There are many beautiful perfume bottles around, and if you enjoy trawling through junk shops and antique markets you may well find some beautiful secondhand perfume bottles to use. Old perfume bottles, especially those that are collector's items, can be expensive, but with luck you'll find some that are beautiful without having a large price tag. Do check the bottle over to make sure that the lid fits securely and that there are no obvious flaws in the glass.

No matter how old it is, it is imperative that you wash the bottle to remove all traces of old perfume. To do this, wash the bottle in hot soapy water, then rinse it at least twice in clean hot water. Leave it to dry naturally, then smell the inside of the bottle to make sure any aromatic remains have disappeared. If you can still detect a trace of aroma, rinse the bottle with a solution of rubbing alcohol – such as surgical spirit or isopropyl alcohol – and hot water. Do a final rinse in hot water and leave to drain and dry.

Whether you decide to use bottles with spray attachments or roll-on bottles, sourcing what you want and in quantities that are manageable can often be a daunting task. If antique markets aren't your choice, then the internet is an excellent place to start your search for new perfume bottles and containers.

Googling 'perfume bottles' is likely to bring up sites that sell perfumes, but if you enter 'perfume containers' or 'perfume packaging' the search should return a list of perfume packaging suppliers. However, it won't take long for you to discover that the biggest choice of bottles in terms of designs and sizes come from suppliers in the USA or China.

You'll also find that buying in small quantities increases the price of bottles, but buying in bulk (10,000 units upwards) makes prices far more reasonable. However, unless you've decided to take a giant step into perfume manufacture, buying in bulk isn't what you need (yet!).

When you find suppliers with reasonably priced, decently sized, perfectly shaped bottles that are sold in individual units or small quantities, ask if they will provide you with a sample if you plan to buy several bottles. If you're buying glass bottles, then a sample may not be necessary, but if you're buying plastic ones, then you should test the bottle to make sure that it is suitable for your perfumed products.

Testing your bottles

Testing simply requires you to fill the bottle with a perfume product, then leave it for three to six months to ensure there is no warping or other degradation of the bottle. Of course you may not have a six-month window available in which to test your bottles; in this case make sure you choose a material that is known to be reliable.

Types of plastic perfume bottles

There are several different types of plastic, such as HDPE (high-density polyethylene), LDPE (low-density polyethylene), HPPE (high-pressure polyethylene), PVC (polyvinyl chloride) and PET (polyethylene terephthalate) that you can choose from.

Some of these bottle materials are suitable for certain perfume products while others aren't, due to the small molecular structure of some perfume oils migrating into the plastics, causing them to buckle and warm. A heavily diluted perfume product such as eau de toilette or eau fraîche is fine for bottles such as these, but stronger parfums may cause a problem, which is why these are usually packaged in glass.

Use this checklist to help you decide which materials are suitable for your perfumes. If in doubt, ask your supplier and be prepared to test your bottle.

Packaging Material	Parfum	Eau de Parfum	Eau de Toilette	Eau Fraîche
HDPE	Yes	Yes	Yes	Yes
LDPE	No	No	No	Yes
HPPE	No	No	No	No
PVC	No	No	No	Yes
PET	Yes	Yes	Yes	Yes
Aluminium	Yes	Yes	Yes	Yes
Lacquer-lined Steel/Tin	Yes	Yes	Yes	Yes
Glass	Yes	Yes	Yes	Yes

Bottle closures

Once you've found the size, shape and style of bottle you want, you'll then need to make a decision about closures. Be warned that when you buy a bottle, it's unlikely that the bottle lid or other attachment is included as part of the purchase. This isn't always the case – sometimes regular plastic screw lids are included – but if you want more specialist closures, then you normally have to buy these separately.

While most websites will guide you through the appropriately sized closures, it is useful to know how these are measured so that you can have the freedom of buying from other suppliers with the peace of mind that they will fit your bottles.

When buying roll-on bottles, the roller ball and lid will always be included with the bottle.

Spray closures

The styles of closure for a perfume spray differ in terms of material and colour. Spray attachments typically have three areas you need to focus on: the collar of the spray attachment, the spray itself (the bit you push down to release a spray of liquid) and the lid that covers the spray. Each of these can be available in metal or plastic.

Closure neck sizes

All bottle necks are measured in size. There are two sizes for each bottle: the diameter and the depth. If you buy the correct diameter but not the correctly sized depth, the spray attachment will not fit your bottle.

If you see a lid described as 24/410, this means that the neck size is 24 (24mm in diameter) and the depth is 410mm. Be warned: you'll be able to buy lids that may fit the neck of the bottle in terms of diameter, but may be too long or too short to screw on properly. Check the resources section on page 153 for details of packaging suppliers.

Storing your perfume

As with all cosmetics, perfume likes to be kept somewhere cool and, preferably, dark, as heat and light cause perfume to deteriorate. Perfumes in dark-glass or aluminium bottles will automatically be kept in the dark because the bottles' solid walls prevent light penetration. Perfumes in transparent glass bottles need to be kept away from direct sunlight – so don't store them on your window sill.

Perfume is like wine and once opened and exposed to the air, it will start the slow process of oxidisation. While this may not become apparent for many years, the lovely boost of wonderful fresh scent will gradually deteriorate and the perfume may become darker in colour. Keep perfume bottles tightly stoppered. Always keep the lid on so that the likelihood of air transference is reduced.

Shelf life of your perfume

If stored properly, perfume will last several hundred years. Many vials and jars of perfumes have been found in Egyptian tombs aeons after they were locked away, yet the aroma is as good and strong today as it was thousands of years ago, when it was made.

Regardless of how they are stored, however, perfumes will change slightly as they age. Molecules evolve and transform, albeit not necessarily detectably by our sense of smell. Oils such as patchouli mature with age, for example, and an old bottle of wonderfully syrupy patchouli will have far more depth and character than a fresh, raw, recently distilled one. The maturing process will continue even after the patchouli has been blended with other oils.

TO CONCLUDE...

- Choosing suitable perfume bottles can be time-consuming. You must decide not only the size and style of the bottles you want, but also make sure that the material is suitable for your perfumes. Having chosen the bottles, you then need to choose appropriate lids or spray attachments, making sure that the ones you want will fit your bottles.
- Storing your perfume in a cool, dark place can help to keep it fresh and prevent the aroma from fading.

NAMING YOUR PERFUME

Another exciting part of making your perfume is to think of a name. I know that this can sometimes be the longest and most taxing element of making your perfume, and I have lost hours trying to come up with the perfect name for my perfect fragrance.

Regardless of what you end up naming your perfume, you must do a little research to make sure that the name hasn't been used by anyone else (start by Googling it), that it isn't offensive to any race, religion, sex or creed, and that it doesn't have an alternative meaning that may be unnecessarily shocking, teasingly humorous or embarrassing.

Don't necessarily reject any names you initially come up with; create a list, then make a decision, possibly saving some of the rejected names for future perfumes. While names such as Knowing, Wrapping, Chaos and Fahrenheit may not grab you at first glance, they were once on someone's list – and now they grace our perfume shelves as well-known names. Below I've listed a random sample of some brand-name perfumes and suggested their intended impact on us, the consumers.

Foreign-language names

Giving a perfume a French name adds a romantic element to the perfume. Possibly translating the same words into German, Swedish or Russian may remove a little of the tender-loving edge.

Calling a perfume something very straightforward, such as such as 'Little Black Dress', can instantly sound enthralling when translated into French – La Petite Robe Noir (Guerlain). It would be brave to call your perfume after a piece of furniture, and yet Cuir Ottoman (Parfum d'Empire) sounds perfectly acceptable.

Do be careful if you plan to use a different language, however. Do some research as to how the word or phrase may be translated in other languages. Magie Noir (Lancôme), for instance, translates to 'Black Magic', which is also the name of a well-known box of chocolates. One of my students named her perfume in Swahili after the name of a tree. When another student translated the name from Swahili into her mother tongue, she found out that it meant 'murderer' – not what was intended at all!

Moody names

Happy (Clinique), and Joy (Jean Patou) conjure up good feelings and suggest that by wearing the perfume, these emotions and sentiments will be bestowed upon you. Bearing that in mind, Arrogance pour Femme (Schiapparelli), Wicked (Bijan) and Envy (Gucci) make interesting choices...

Colourful names

Possibly harnessing the idea of colour therapy, Red (the colour symbolic of danger) has been used in many perfume names, such as Red Delicious Men (Donna Karan), Burberry Brit Red (Burberry), Lacoste Red (Lacoste) and oddly, Red Door (Elizabeth Arden).

Many perfumes have colours in their name. These range from the more obviously tempting, such as Dazzling Gold (Estée Lauder), Green Energy (Givenchy), Blue Marine (Pierre Cardin) and White Diamonds (Elizabeth Taylor) to the perhaps less temptingly named White Shoulders (again by Elizabeth Arden) and Grey Flannel (Geoffrey Beene).

Historical/literary names

Aramis (Estée Lauder) is named after one of the fictional characters in Dumas' *The Three Musketeers,* while the perfume house, Histoires de Parfums, has perfumes called 1725, 1740, 1804, 1826 and so forth, each dedicated to characters who were inspirational at that time.

Celebrity/design house names

Many perfume and design houses have a flagship perfume named after the company or a designer such as Marc Jacobs (Marc Jacobs), Oscar (Oscar de la Renta) and CK One (Calvin Klein). Celebrity endorsement of perfumes leads consumers to believe they are buying a little piece of the celebrity in the hope that they can share a similar lifestyle. The model Kate Moss is one of the few celebrities to have a perfume named after her as well as being endorsed by her. Other celebrity-endorsed perfumes include Sexy Darling (Kylie Minogue) and Beautiful (Sarah Jessica Parker). Etat Libre d'Orange has a perfume called Tom of Finland but I've yet to discover who Tom is or was!

Descriptive names

To save you wondering what a perfume smells like, many perfume houses name their products after a perfume's key aromatic ingredients. Jo Malone products are good examples of this, with Dark Amber and Ginger Lily, White Jasmine and Mint, and Orange Blossom and Honey, to name just three. Others include Tobacco Vanille (Tom Ford), White Rose (Floris) and Night Scented Jasmine (Floris). Nothing adventurous here, but good, honest, what-you-see-is-what-you-get names.

Adventurous and obscure names

Calling a perfume Poison (Dior) was a bold move, and one that certainly worked, as is White Linen (Estée Lauder), which may conjure up clean clothes but isn't instantly representative of an aroma. Both Cool Water and Hot Water (Davidoff) are interesting choices, especially since water, regardless of its temperature, has no smell.

I'm still baffled, but rather in awe of a perfume named What About Adam (Joop!). (Who was this Adam and what about him?)

Both Chanel and Carolina Herrera, among others, have taken something simple and made it theirs. Chanel has a range of numbered perfumes: Chanel No 5, No 18, No 19 and No 22. Similarly, Carolina Herrera has taken the number 212 and made it hers, with 212 Sexy, 212 Men, 212 Splash, 212 VIP, 212 H20 and just plain 212 on its own.

TO CONCLUDE...

- The name you choose for your perfume needs to have some thought behind it to ensure that it isn't offensive or embarrassing if translated into another language or taken out of context.
- Don't be shy and don't reject names that you like because they don't initially seem glamorous or catchy.
- Stop and think about the names of many popular perfumes. They may sound weird if taken out of context, yet within the world of perfume, they sit perfectly comfortably and we don't even give them a second thought.

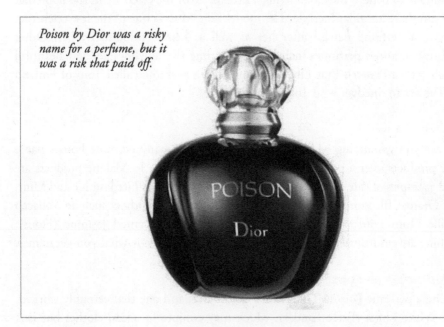

Poison by Dior was a risky name for a perfume, but it was a risk that paid off.

DESCRIBING YOUR PERFUME

Being able to describe a perfume so that it sounds sufficiently tempting, delicious and mouth-watering to entice anyone to beg you for a sample is of paramount importance if you wish others to wear your perfume. But unless you have an advertising budget that allows you to shout out to the world about your product, the only way others can appreciate your perfume without physically smelling it is by the use of carefully chosen words.

Describing a perfume is difficult. Describing the smell of foods is much easier, since the aroma of food stuffs is more familiar to us. The smell of cooking bacon, fish, sprouts, roast potatoes and chicken korma can be imagined without the food being prepared in our presence, and yet the smell of musk, amber, tonka bean, violets, jasmine, hyacinth and so on is not as apparent in our imagination.

Carefully chosen descriptive words help to place the aromas and sharpen our senses. You could describe your perfume as 'nice and fruity', for example, but 'fruity with a hint of gardenia' is more appealing.

Don't stop there; take it further with 'fruity with a hint of gardenia entwined with a herbaceous layer', or, better still, 'fruity with a hint of gardenia entwined with a herbaceous layer yielding to an undertone of amber'... or even 'fruity with a hint of gardenia entwined with a herbaceous layer yielding to an undertone of amber infused with a floral sweetness of vanilla and honey'.

Keep building on the descriptive words without totally confusing your audience. Your description has to be imaginable or you will lose them at the herbaceous layer stage.

A perfect description for your perfume could run along the lines of the following:

'A sparkling zest of pink grapefruit is tamed with the delicate sweetness of orange blossom, quenched with a generous bouquet of gardenia to awaken your senses. Energetic green spices burst in with a layer of herbaceous brilliance to enliven and rejuvenate. A heady cocktail of patchouli and vetiver seduced by an amber infusion of vanilla and honey blossom leave a sweet aftertaste that lingers and leaves you wanting more.'

Now *that* sounds like a perfume I'd like to try right now! The description has hooked me in, leaving me desperate to try some.

Keep a portfolio of descriptive words you can use to bring your perfumes to life. Here are a few to start you off.

Airy	Animalic	Balsamic
Bitter	Camphorous	Cheap
Citrusy	Clean	Creamy
Damp	Dry	Ethereal
Fat	Fecal	Fizzy
Floral	Fresh	Fruity
Grassy	Green	Herbaceous
Inky	Invigorating	Light
Lively	Metallic	Mild
Milky	Mossy	Musky
Oaky	Peppery	Powdery
Pungent	Rejuvenating	Resinous
Reviving	Sharp	Smoky
Sour	Spicy	Spicy
Sulphuraceous	Swampy	Sweet
Syrupy	Tart	Thin
Watery	Woody	Zingy

Labelling your perfume

When giving a bottle of your perfume to someone else, you should think about labelling it just to make sure they know what they've been given. If you don't have sticky labels to hand, or don't want to stick a label on the container, then tie it around the neck with a pretty ribbon or piece of raffia.

The label should at least tell the recipient what the product is – parfum, eau de parfum, eau de toilette or eau fraîche – so that she has an idea of the strength of the perfume and therefore hopefully how much to apply. It should also include the perfume name. If you plan on selling your perfume, the EU Cosmetic Regulations have strict guidelines on what needs to go on your labels.

As consumers, we ought to know how to unravel the information on a label so that we can understand and appreciate what it is trying to convey. Because it is difficult to print such a wealth of information directly onto a bottle, this information is usually printed on the box or on a leaflet tucked inside the perfume box.

Information you'd expect to find on a box of perfume
Every perfume formulation is considered to be a secret. Imagine being able to work out the precise ingredients from a label. There would be so many attempted copies of Chanel No 5 that the real Chanel No 5 would no longer be special.

For this reason, the ingredients in a perfume blend are exempt from disclosure and are simply listed as 'Parfum' (or you may see it listed as 'Fragrance'). The individual components of the perfume blend do not have to be listed separately, which allows the formula to remain a secret. Other non-aromatic perfume ingredients are listed, though, such as the dilutant, colourings and any preservatives.

Example of a perfume ingredients list
Alcohol Denat This is the ingredient (denatured alcohol) used to dilute the perfume. As it is the largest in volume, it is listed first in the ingredients list.

Parfum (Fragrance) The perfume blend: a combination of 'secret' perfume ingredients.

Linalool, Limonene, Geraniol, Benzyl Salicylate, Benzyl Alcohol, and Benzyl Benzoate These compounds occur naturally in essential oils and can be reproduced synthetically to emulate a natural aroma in fragrance oils. There are 16 of these compounds, also known as allergens, that can occur in essential oils. Each needs to be listed if the relevant perfume essential oil has been used as part of the perfume blend.

Amyl Cinnamal and Hexyl Cinnamal These are synthetic compounds used to emulate a natural aroma in fragrance oils. As well as the 16 allergens mentioned above, a further ten may be found in perfume fragrance oils, and these will need to be listed as well if the relevant perfume fragrance oil has been used as part of the perfume blend. Anyone who suffers an allergic reaction to a particular allergen will want to know whether the perfume contains these allergens or not. This will allow them to make an informed decision as to whether they should buy and wear the perfume.

CI14720 (Red 4) and CI14190 (Yellow 9)
Cosmetic-grade colours approved for use in cosmetics and perfumes.

TO CONCLUDE...
- If you aren't going to sell your perfume then how you label it is down to you.
- It is advisable, however, that you label it so that you, and anyone you give it to, know what the bottle contains. Knowing how strong the perfume is will help you decide how much you should apply without drowning yourself in the smell.

HOW TO WEAR YOUR PERFUME

You could take the advice of Coco Chanel, who said you should only wear perfume where you want to be kissed! However, most of us either spray the bottle over our décolletage (chest and neck) area and onto our wrists, or dab it onto our wrists. Traditionally, perfume was worn behind the ears, although I'm not certain many of us take the effort to place our perfume there these days.

Contrary to what we're often told, do not rub your perfumed wrists together, as this will only serve to warm up the perfume, causing it to evaporate faster. Try a little experiment. Spray an equal amount of perfume onto each of your wrists. Allow the perfume on each wrist to dry. Leave one wrist alone but rub the other onto a section of bare skin – the crook of your elbow or onto your leg. Smell each of your wrists straight away and then smell them again 15 minutes later. The wrist that you didn't rub should smell stronger. This is because the rubbed wrist was warmer, causing the perfume to evaporate faster than the cooler wrist.

Where to wear your perfume

Perfume should be applied to your pulse points, such as in the crook of your elbow and backs of your knees, your wrist, neck, ankles and cleavage. These areas are your warm areas and will allow the perfume to release its scent gradually.

Remember that warm air rises, so don't only apply your perfume to your neck. Dotting it behind your knees or even on the tops of your feet will help you to enjoy the aroma for longer.

Most perfumes are fragrance oils diluted in alcohol and will evaporate from your skin over time, releasing the different aromas at different stages. It is the temperature of your skin and where you wear your perfume that will have an impact on how long it lasts and even the way it smells.

Where the blood is closer to the surface of the skin – e.g. your neck, wrists and throat – the fragrance will be warmer and evaporate faster than perfume in cooler skin areas.

Perfume carried about your person, but not actually on your body, generally lasts longer because it remains cooler. To wear perfume in this way, consider spraying it onto your clothes, hair or onto a cotton-wool ball that you can tuck into your clothing.

Hair perfume

This is a perfect way of wearing perfume, but not one that many of us utilise. Gently spray a waft of perfume into your hair, being very careful not to get it in your eyes. Roll-on perfume bottles can be used to roll perfume on to the hair shaft.

Google 'hair perfume' and you'll be surprised how many hairdressers have joined forces with perfume houses to bring out their signature hair-perfume fragrances!

How much to wear?

How much perfume you wear is a personal choice, but rather than douse your friends and colleagues in a cloud that leaves them tasting it when they swallow, you should aim to wear just enough to draw their attention, heighten their senses and leave them interested.

Keep your perfume floating in your personal space rather than drenching the room as soon as you walk into it. You want others to be curious and fascinated – not keen to find fresh air!

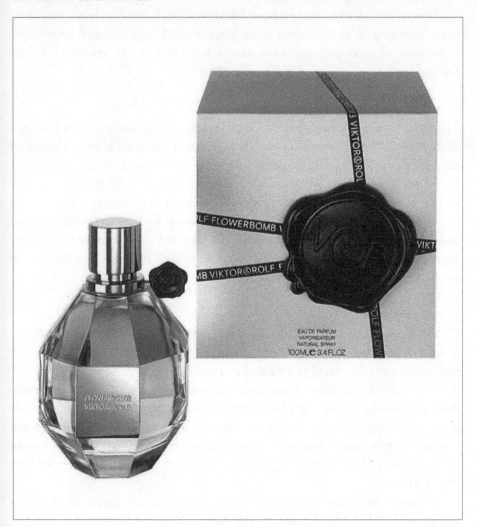

THE POWER OF SMELL

People often believe that their perfume has lost its aroma, but before you reach for the bottle to apply more, ask a friend if he or she can smell the perfume on you. More often than not, the answer will be yes: the aroma is still easily detectable.

This is because the 'smell receiving' part your brain has already engaged with the aroma of our perfume, registered any actions it may be required to take and then categorised it as a familiar, safe smell, with no further action necessary. The brain then moves on to other smells, seemingly ignoring the perfume – leading you to believe you can no longer smell it.

Having a break from that perfume for a few weeks is sensible. In the very short term, breathing in and smelling fresh, clean air will help to 'reset' your brain's registration of your perfume. Let's have a brief look at the chemistry behind this concept.

A powerful sense

The word 'olfactory' comes from the Latin *olfactare,* which means to sniff at, and *olfacere,* which means to smell. Our olfactory nerves continually renew themselves throughout our lifetime. This means that smells you enjoyed in puberty may not be the smells that please you as an adult. Perfumes you thought were a must-have in your teens may not be the perfumes you choose to buy ten years later.

The sense of smell is powerful and uncontrollable. We have the ability to detect and register over 10,000 different smells. The power of smell tends to be the least-appreciated of the five senses – unless you're an animal, in which case the sense of smell can be a matter of life or death.

How do we smell?

All smells enter the body via the nostrils. Located in our nostrils are turbinate bones that swirl the air around the nostril cavity so that every bit of air passes over the smell organs. We smell as we breathe in and out of our nostrils.

This part of the lining in the nose accommodates special nerve cells whose fibres connect directly through the olfactory nerves to the brain. The olfactory bulb is part of the brain's limbic system, an area associated with memory and emotion – which is why smells instantly trigger memories and change people's moods. This chemistry is the stuff that perfumers dream of being able to control with their perfume.

Olfactory nerves are made up of minute fibres whose tips are covered in tiny waving hairs called cilia. As the air circulates in the nostrils, it passes over and latches on to the cilia. It is then that a signal is sent to the brain in order to register the smell. Different nerve endings register different smells – which are recognised by their molecular shape and chemical nature.

Why do we smell?

Whenever your brain detects an odour it registers whether any action needs to take place. For example, if it detects an aroma from food, it kick-starts the production of digestive juices needed to break down and absorb the food when it is eaten. If the aroma detected isn't from food, then possibly the smell is a there to alert you into running, fighting, or even to trigger a desire to have sex. Many perfumes contain levels of pheromone-like substances, and these perfumes are advertised as making you feel sensual or sexy.

Different perceptions of the same smell

Everyone distinguishes aromas slightly differently. The smell of violet may take some on an imaginary journey to a sweet-shop reminiscent of parma violet sweets, while others may simply smell violet and have no trigger of any emotion or memory.

Perfumes are complex mixtures of many aromas. Two people smelling the same perfume may notice different scents. One may claim to detect the aroma of vanilla, while the other might find that the scent of pineapple is more apparent. Neither is wrong; it's just that each person has connected with a different element of the same perfume.

TO CONCLUDE...

- Wear your perfume on your skin or your clothing. The warmer parts of your skin will cause the perfume to evaporate into the air, making it more noticeable but also causing it to disappear faster.
- If you feel your perfume has lost its smell, ask someone else for their opinion before applying more. Take a break from wearing the perfume to allow your brain into 'deregister' the smell.
- Different people may detect different aroma components in your perfume. The more layers in your perfume, the more interesting and memorable it will be.

CHAPTER 9

Making Tinctures and Infusions

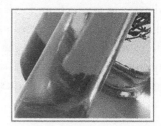

Extracting the aromatic essence from herbs and flowers into a liquid that you can use as part of your perfume-making involves making a tincture or an infusion. This does not require any special equipment and can be done at home.

Being able to make a tincture or infusion opens up a whole new world when it comes to making perfume. Any tangible, solid item that has an aroma can be infused in oil or alcohol in order to extract its aroma and capture it in a liquid. You can then use this liquid as part of your perfume blend.

Making a tincture

Tinctures are a mixture of alcohol and plant material. The plant material is the aromatic part of the plant such as rose petals, lavender heads and stalks, herb leaves, frankincense or myrrh tears, amber or benzoin resins, juniper berries, vanilla pods, cinnamon sticks and cloves.

Alcohol extracts the aroma from the plant and captures it in the alcohol. Suitable alcohols to use are ethyl alcohol, isopropyl rubbing alcohol, denatured alcohol, perfumers' alcohol or vodka. The alcohol should not be consumed; it is for perfumed topical skin application only. The process used in making a tincture is called maceration.

How to make a tincture

You will need the following equipment:

- Pestle and mortar
- Glass jar with lid in which to develop the tincture
- Fine sieve, muslin or filter paper
- Clean bottle with lid to store the tincture (dark glass is preferable)

Ingredients
- 3–4 handfuls of your chosen plant material (or combination of plant materials)
- Sufficient alcohol to cover the plant material

1. Chop or grind the plant material into small pieces – the smaller the pieces, the better the tincture.

2. Put the crushed plant material into the glass jar and cover it with alcohol so that the plant material is submerged. Ideally, fill the jar with the plant material and then fill up to the neck of the jar with alcohol. This minimises the amount of air in the jar.

3. Put the lid on to the jar and give the mixture a shake.

4. Place the jar in a cool cupboard for two weeks. Shake the jar daily to mix the plant material with the alcohol.

5. At the end of the two-week period, strain the liquid through a piece of muslin, fine mesh sieve or filter paper. The filter papers used for coffee machines make useful tincture filters.

6. Pour the liquid into a dark glass bottle, then label the bottle with the date and the contents.

To use the tincture as a perfume

Place a little tincture on your skin and smell it. If it isn't strong enough, you can repeat the process above using a fresh set of plant material. If it is strong enough, then either wear it as it is, or blend it with your perfume oils.

Once blended with perfume oils, treat the tincture as part of the perfume oil base and add further dilutant according to the required strength of your final perfumed product.

Making an infusion

An infusion is similar to a tincture, but instead of alcohol, a carrier oil is used. The final result is a scented oil that can be applied directly to the skin. The infusion can be used as part of your perfume blend, but it will make your perfume a little greasy. Suitable oils include jojoba, avocado, sweet almond, fractionated coconut and rice bran oil. Infusions can be used as part of a solid perfume base.

How to make an infusion
You will need the following equipment:

- Pestle and mortar
- Glass jar with lid in which to develop the infusion
- Fine sieve or muslin
- Clean bottle with lid to store the infusion (dark glass is preferable)

Ingredients
- 3–4 handfuls of chosen plant material (or combination of plant materials)
- Sufficient oil to cover the plant material

1. Chop or grind the plant material into small pieces – the smaller the pieces, the better the infusion.

2. Put the crushed plant material into the glass jar and cover with your chosen oil so that the plant material is submerged. Ideally fill the jar with the plant material and then fill up to the neck of the jar with oil to minimise the amount of air in the jar.

3. Put the lid on to the jar and give the mixture a shake.

4. Place the jar on a window-sill for six to eight weeks (or longer if you have the patience).

5. At the end of the eight-week period, strain the oil through a piece of muslin or fine-mesh sieve. You may need to strain the oil twice to remove all traces of plant debris. Using a filter paper for an infusion is not always successful because the oil may be too thick to drip through the paper.

6. Pour the infused oil into a dark glass bottle. Label the bottle with the date and the contents.

An alternative method

It is possible to make a quick infusion by crushing the plant material and adding it to a saucepan. Some plant material scents are destroyed by heat, however, so this method is not recommended for heat-sensitive plants, usually flowers.

1. Pour the oils into the saucepan and place over a low heat, allowing the warmed oils to absorb the aroma from the plant materials.

2. Keep on a low heat for 15–20 minutes and allow to cool before straining.

Using your oil infusion

If the aroma is strong enough, you can use the oil directly on your skin as a scented body oil. If the aroma is not as strong or structured as you would like, use the infusion as part of your perfume blend, further diluting it with oils as necessary.

A little of the perfume oil can be used in a spray perfume if diluted with an appropriate alcohol, but do be aware that this perfume spray with be a little greasy and may mark clothing or anything that it lands on.

Infused oils are ideal as part of a solid perfume.

CHAPTER 10

Making Other Fragranced Products

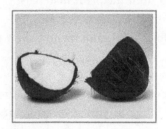

FRAGRANCING YOUR BODY

There are many ways of carrying a delightful aroma on your person without using a perfume. Many perfume houses have introduced other perfumed products to allow you to 'layer' your smell, building perfumed product upon perfumed product. Be careful not to overdo it, though; nobody wants to breathe in and taste your perfume!

The perfume blend you create can also be used in other scented products. The rules of structuring your blend by using top, middle and base notes to give depth, layers and longevity apply, regardless of the product you're making. What changes are the ingredients you use to dilute the perfume blend.

At the end of each section I have suggested six recipes eminently suitable for the perfumed products in question.

Making solid perfumes

Solid perfumes are useful in that they are small and convenient to carry around with you and, because they are solid, they don't spill – although care must be taken not to leave them anywhere hot because they can soften to the point of melting.

Since they aren't sprayed into the air, there is little or no wastage. They moisturise your skin and can be easily rubbed onto most parts of your body.

How to make a solid perfume

This recipe makes approximately 30g of solid perfume. You will need the following equipment:

- Scales
- Heat source (gas, electricity, convection or aga)
- Double boiler (a heatproof jug or bowl placed in a pan of simmering water will do)
- A spoon for stirring
- A lidded container for your solid perfume

Ingredients
- 10g cocoa butter
- 5g wax, such as beeswax, olive wax or jojoba wax (for a slightly softer solid perfume, reduce the wax to 4g)
- 15g carrier oil, such as fractionated coconut, sweet almond, jojoba, avocado or rice bran oil; either a single oil or a combination of the oils mentioned above (for a slightly harder solid perfume, reduce the amount of carrier oil 12g)
- 1-2g of your perfume blend (approximately 30-60 drops)

1. Put the cocoa butter and wax into a heatproof jug or bowl and place the bowl into a shallow pan of hot water. Allow wax and butter to melt, stirring occasionally.

2. When the wax and butter have melted, carefully remove the heatproof jug or bowl from the heat and add the carrier oil/s. Stir well, and add your perfume blend. Stir again to ensure that the blend is thoroughly mixed into the melted wax, butter and oil mix.

3. Pour the cooling mixture into your container but don't put the lid on until the perfume has set. This prevents any steam from evaporating and causing condensation inside the pot.

4. Once the perfume has set, put the lid on and label the pot so that you know what it contains. The shelf life of your solid perfume is two years from the date it was made.

Using your solid perfume

Rub your finger across the solid perfume and then apply it to your pulse points. Solid perfume can also be used anywhere on the body, but please avoid the face and other delicate areas, as perfume oils may be a little too strong for sensitive skin.

Solid perfume recipes

Each of the recipes below makes 60 drops perfume oil – approximately 2g – and can be used as perfume oil in your solid perfume.

Rose Stardom	Vanilla Dreams	Amber Infusion Confusion
4 drops Anise	2 drops Ginger	Create an amber infusion by infusing
25 drops Rose	8 drops Strawberry	amber resin in jojoba oil and including
13 drops Palmarosa	25 drops Vanilla	it as your carrier oil ingredient. Also
2 drops Bay	5 drops Amber	add the following perfume oil blend:
9 drops Rosewood	20 drops Tonka Bean	8 drops Orange
7 drops Benzoin		10 drops White Tea
		35 drops Amber
		3 drops Chocolate
		4 drops Labdanum
Mystique	Fresh Dew	Crushed
10 drops Neroli	12 drops Watermelon	6 drops Petitgrain
6 drops Mandarin	12 drops Lemon Grass	10 drops Juniper Berry
10 drops Peach	9 drops Grass	4 drops Clove
6 drops Blackcurrant	12 drops Bamboo	20 drops Plum
10 drops Pink Pepper	13 drops Honey	15 drops Tuberose
8 drops Honey	2 drops Vetiver	5 drops Patchouli
10 drops Frankincense		

Making scented body oils

Scented body oils are a traditional way of carrying an aroma on your body. They were used as a base for perfume long before perfumers' alcohol, and have the added advantage of moisturising your body, leaving skin silky-smooth.

How to make a scented body oil

This recipe makes approximately 50ml of scented body oil. You will need:

- Scales
- A jug or other container in which to mix the ingredients
- A spoon for stirring
- A lidded bottle

Ingredients
- 50g carrier oil, such as fractionated coconut sweet almond, jojoba, avocado or rice bran oil. The 50g can be a single oil or a combination of oils.
- 2g perfume blend (approximately 60 drops)

1. Pour your chosen carrier oil, or blend of oils, into the mixing jug. Add your perfume blend and stir well.

2. Carefully pour the scented body oil into a bottle and replace the lid. Label the bottle so that you know what it contains. The shelf life of your scented body oil is 12 months from the date it was made.

Using your scented body oil

After a bath or shower, pat your body dry with a towel, then apply a small amount of scented oil. Massage the oil onto your body until it has been absorbed and leaves no greasy residue. Alternatively, apply the oil to your body before bathing, then wash and rinse as usual.

Scented body oil recipes

Each of the recipes below and opposite makes 60 drops of perfume oil – approximately 2g – and can be used as the perfume blend in your body oil.

Morning Glory	Energiser	Humes
15 drops Coconut	15 drops Petitgrain	16 drops Watermelon
10 drops Pomegranate	10 drops Grapefruit	16 drops Salty Sea Dog
20 drops Jasmine	15 drops Bergamot	10 drops Cucumber
8 drops Tuberose	5 drops May Chang	7 drops Champagne
7 drops Ylang-ylang	5 drops Coriander	3 drops Leather
	4 drops Fig Leaf	8 drops Sandalwood
	4 drops Tobacco Leaf	
	2 drops Vetiver	

Merrygold	Soir de Noir	Caprice
7 drops Peppermint	7 drops Lemon	8 drops Cucumber
30 drops Plum	8 drops Blackcurrant	20 drops Mango
3 drops Leather	5 drops Violet	5 drops Frangipani
5 drops Coffee	5 drops Jasmine	7 drops Strawberry
15 drops Vanilla	6 drops Labdanum	5 drops White Tea
5 drops Cherry	2 drops Leather	15 drops Honey
	2 drops Chocolate	
	10 drops Black Tea	
	5 drops Tonka Bean	
	5 drops Benzoin	

Making scented bath oils

It is possible to use your scented body oil as a bath oil; however, bathwater and body oils won't blend. This means that you will have droplets of oil floating around in your bath – and naturally the floor of the bath will become slippery.

In order to make a bath oil that disperses into bathwater, making the entire bath moisturising and skin-softening without the oil droplets, you'll need to include another ingredient: a dispersant.

The dispersant included in the recipe below is polysorbate 80. Polysorbate 80 is derived from olive oil and sorbitol, an artificial sweetener. Its role is to disperse your bath oil with the bathwater so that the result is a milky, moisturising liquid, but not one that leaves a greasy film or has oil droplets. Your bath may still be slippery, though, so please take care when stepping in and out it.

How to make a scented bath oil

This recipe makes approximately 100ml scented bath oil. The shelf life of your bath oil is 12 months from the date it was made. You will need the following equipment:

- Scales
- A jug or other container in which to mix the ingredients
- A spoon for stirring
- A lidded bottle

Ingredients
- 20g polysorbate 80
- 78g grapeseed oil or sweet almond oil
- 2–3g perfume oil blend (60–90 drops)
- 2g perfume blend (approximately 60 drops)

1. Pour the polysorbate 80 and the grapeseed or sweet almond oil into the mixing jug. Add your perfume blend and stir well.

2. Carefully pour the scented bath oil into a bottle and replace the lid. Label the bottle so that you know what it contains.

Using your scented bath oil

The bottle you have made holds enough for six baths. Pour one-sixth of the scented bath oil into warm, running bathwater and swoosh it through the bathwater to disperse.

Scented bath oil recipes

Each of the recipes below makes 60 drops of perfume oil – approximately 2g – and can be used as the perfume oil in your scented bath oil.

Amourama	Snazzle	Mediterranean Radiance
50 drops Rose	8 drops Lemon	25 drops Neroli
2 drops Champagne	10 drops Apple	8 drops Orange
4 drops Amber	4 drops Black Pepper	4 drops Lime
4 drops Patchouli	15 drops Bamboo	5 drops Geranium
	10 drops Coriander	10 drops Lavender
	3 drops Vetiver	8 drops Labdanum
Tia d'Été	**Emerald Blue**	**Sweet Lime Summer**
15 drops Lime	6 drops Grapefruit	5 drops Anise
15 drops Mandarin	5 drops Clary Sage	25 drops Lime
10 drops Basil	6 drops Cucumber	5 drops Bay
12 drops Lemon Grass	6 drops Coriander	5 drops Gardenia
8 drops Coffee	10 drops Hyacinth	8 drops Rose
	5 drops Lily of the Valley	5 drops Frangipani
	2 drops Rosemary	7 drops Honey
	10 drops Tobacco Leaf	
	10 drops Oakmoss	

FRAGRANCING YOUR HOME

Just as your handmade perfumed products can make you smell lovely, you can also make products that help your home smell gorgeous, too. When choosing which home fragrance products to make, decide whether you want a permanent aroma, in which case you will want to make potpourri, scented beads or a room diffuser, or whether you want to choose when to release the aroma into your room, in which case a room spray is more appropriate.

Making a scented room diffuser

Room diffusers have become popular in the last few years. A room diffuser set comprises a bottle containing a scented liquid and several reed diffuser sticks. Reed sticks draw up the liquid, rather like a straw. Once the scented liquid has saturated the stick, it evaporates into the air, throwing its scent into the room.

Depending on the strength of the scented liquid and the structure of the perfume oil, your diffuser can last for six months or so until it needs replenishing.

The key ingredient to make the reed diffuser sticks work particularly well is dipropylene glycol. Dipropylene glycol is used extensively in the perfume industry – you may remember that it is an ingredient in perfumers' alcohol (see page 93). As well as being odourless and colourless, its main advantage is that it slows the evaporation of molecules, therefore making your perfume last longer.

The same functionality is important for our reed diffusers. The dipropylene glycol helps to slow the evaporation of the perfume blend. This is especially important because the diffuser perfume blend is contained in a bottle that doesn't have a lid, so it will 'want' to evaporate faster than a perfume.

As well as dipropylene glycol, perfume oil is also diluted with isopropyl myristate, but cyclomethicone could be used instead.

How to make a scented room diffuser

The reason this recipe calls for a wide-based bottle is because, once the reed sticks are inserted into the bottle, it can become a little top-heavy. Wide-based bottles are less likely to topple over than smaller based bottles. You will need the following equipment:

- Scales
- A jug or other container in which to mix the ingredients
- A spoon for stirring
- A wide-based bottle

Ingredients
- 10g dipropylene glycol
- 50g isopropyl myristate
- 6–10g perfume oil blend (approximately 180–300 drops)

1. Pour the dipropylene glycol, isopropyl myristate and your perfume blend into the mixing jug and stir well.

2. Carefully pour the scented diffuser oil into the wide-based bottle so that it comes about halfway up the bottle. Pour any excess into a lidded bottle and use it to top up the diffuser bottle as necessary. Don't forget to label the lidded bottle.

Using your scented room diffuser
Tuck the diffuser bottle somewhere out of the way in the room you wish to scent. Insert 5 diffuser sticks into the bottle. It will take up to 24 hours for the perfumed liquid to rise up the sticks and to start to evaporate into the room.

Room diffuser recipes

Wild Island	Summer Tropics	Bear Hug
20 drops Clove	20 drops Frangipani	25 drops Petitgrain
80 drops Rose	20 drops Lime	25 drops Orange
100 drops Frangipani	20 drops Pineapple	10 drops Lemon
50 drops Patchouli	100 drops Coconut	15 drops Lime
	20 drops Amber	50 drops Lavender
	20 drops Honey	50 drops Grapefruit
		35 drops Rosewood
Ice Ice Baby	**JB**	**Mellifera**
70 drops Peppermint	50 drops Bergamot	35 drops Lilac
90 drops Bergamot	20 drops Basil	30 drops Lily of the Valley
90 drops Orange	20 drops Bay	25 drops Lavender
	55 drops Jasmine	45 drops Heather
	30 drops Patchouli	15 drops Tuberose
	20 drops Cedar	50 drops Vanilla
		45 drops Honey

Making scented potpourri

Potpourri is a mixture of scented petals and herbs that you place in a bowl or a dish and leave on a shelf in a room. The smell gradually fills the room with a gentle aroma. Please make sure it doesn't look edible, though, and isn't mistaken for a bowl of snacks!

Potpourri ingredients

- Use an assortment of natural plant materials for your potpourri. Flower petals, such as rose petals, lavender heads, jasmine petals, make scented and attractive additions. Home-grown herbs and scented leaves such as lemon verbena, Lemon Grass, bay leaves and rosemary are useful, while fir cones, small sticks and other eye-catching foliage help give potpourri visual appeal.
- Use herbs and spices that look attractive, such as cloves, cinnamon sticks, vanilla beans and nutmeg. Leave some of the spices whole, but remove some and crush them in a pestle and mortar to release their aroma. The crushed herbs and spices can be used as part of the potpourri mix.
- Dried fruit peel such as orange, lime, lemon and grapefruit can be included in your mix. Add a little of the relevant essential oil to the dried peel to boost its aroma.
- Orris root powder is an especially useful ingredient in potpourri because it works as a fixative, slowing the evaporation of perfume oils exposed to the air. The temptation is to add more perfume oil, but you want your potpourri to be dry rather than damp to prevent it from going mucky.

You'll need to weigh your potpourri mixture if you wish to be precise about the amount of perfume blend to use. Since this isn't being rubbed onto your body, the amount doesn't have to be exact and you can add as much as you wish – providing you don't make the mixture too damp.

If you want to be more precise, however, then work on adding your perfume blend at a maximum of 10 per cent – i.e. for every 10g potpourri, use a maximum of 1g or 30 drops of your perfume blend. Be aware that heavier items, such as fir cones, need not be weighed;just weigh the leaves, petals, spices, herbs and other plant material that will absorb the perfume blend.

How to make scented potpourri

Your potpourri will have an indefinite shelf life, providing it is not damp. You will need the following equipment:

- 1 large bowl for mixing your potpourri
- A spoon for mixing
- 1 decorative bowl for displaying your potpourri
- Perfume oil blend
- A sealable bag in which to store excess potpourri

1. Choose which petals, herbs, spices and other plant material you wish to use. Only use dry items – if the products are damp, place them on waxed paper or newspaper and leave them somewhere warm and dry until they are crisp with no signs of damp at all.

2. Place the items in a glass or ceramic bowl and gradually drop your perfume oil onto them. If using orris powder, mix the perfume blend with the orris powder first, then stir the orris powder into the plant material.

Using your scented potpourri

Give the bowl a shake to help release the smells. Your potpourri mixture may need topping up with perfume oils from time to time.

Be careful not to allow your new potpourri to come into contact with furniture and surfaces, as it may leave a mark.

Potpourri mixture can also be placed in muslin squares or bags and hung in wardrobes. Don't allow them to touch the clothing, however, in case the bag is oily and leaves a mark on your clothes.

Potpourri recipes

Each of the recipes below makes 60 drops perfume oil – approximately 2g – and can be used as the perfume oil to scent approximately 20g potpourri mix. Remember to blend your perfume oils with a little orris powder to fix them.

Petal Power	Woodland Haven	Inspire
50 drops Rose	10 drops Black Tea	10 drops Mandarin
4 drops Clove	20 drops Juniper Berry	30 drops Lavender
6 drops Benzoin	10 drops Violet	12 drops Sandalwood
	10 drops Cedar	8 drops Patchouli
	10 drops Patchouli	
Spiced Passion	**Please Ami**	**Virtue**
4 drops Cinnamon	10 drops Orange	12 drops Lemon
8 drops Clove	20 drops Rose	35 drops Lavender
12 drops Pink Pepper	5 drops Clove	10 drops Clary Sage
4 drops Ginger	15 drops Rosewood	3 drops Vetiver
22 drops Honey	10 drops Amber	
10 drops Patchouli		

Making scented beads

Scented beads are small plastic beads that absorb and hold a whopping great 30 per cent of their weight in perfume oil! They tend to be stronger than potpourri, so they can be used in smaller quantities while still fragrancing a large area. Because the beads are small, they do need to be contained either in either a bowl or small bag.

How to make scented beads

The shelf life of aroma beads is for as long as you're prepared to keep topping them up with another dose of fragrance oil. You will need the following equipment:

- A lidded jar
- A small bowl or cloth bag with drawstring

Ingredients
- 20g aroma beads
- 6g perfume blend

1. Put your unscented aroma beads into the jar.

2. Add your perfume blend and put the lid on the jar.

3. Give the jar a good shake so that the beads are coated in the perfume blend.

4. Leave for 24 hours to allow the beads to soak up the perfume oil. If, after 24 hours, there is still some perfume oil residue in the jar, add a few more beads to soak it up.

Using your scented beads

Place your scented beads in a bowl or a small drawstring bag. They can be replenished with more perfume oils once the smell has faded. Bags of beads can be hung in your wardrobe, placed in your underwear drawer or put in your trainers or boots. They can also be used to fragrance your car by hanging a little bag off the rearview mirror (but please don't let the bag obscure your vision). Alternatively, place them in the car's clean ashtray and leave the ashtray ajar to allow the smell to emanate.

Put a few of your scented beads in your vacuum cleaner so that it blows out scented air rather than dust-smelling air. The easiest way to place these in your Hoover is by – yes, you guessed it – hoovering them up!

Other suggestions include sewing scented beads into stuffed toys, hiding them in silk flower arrangements, including them with other potpourri items, putting a few in coat pockets, in a small drawstring bag in a pillowcase, in your linen cupboard – and so on!

Scented beads recipes

Each of the recipes below makes 60 drops perfume oil – approximately 2g – and can be used as the perfume oil in your scented beads mix. This is sufficient to fragrance approximately 7g scented beads. If you wish to scent 20g beads, simply multiply the amounts given below by three.

Bacbac	Are We There Yet?	Zuzz
10 drops Eucalyptus	20 drops Peppermint	15 drops Neroli
10 drops Rosemary	10 drops Ginger	10 drops Mandarin
30 drops Lavender	20 drops Coriander	20 drops Hyacinth
10 drops Frankincense	10 drops Amber	10 drops Ylang-ylang
		5 drops Honey
Nooshoo	**Hush**	**Harmony**
20 drops Bergamot	15 drops Petitgrain	9 drops Bergamot
10 drops Salty Sea Dog	5 drops Chamomile	9 drops Orange
10 drops Cucumber	20 drops Lemon Grass	10 drops Fig
15 drops Lilac	10 drops Labdanum	15 drops Mango
4 drops Oakmoss	10 drops Vanilla	7 drops Sandalwood
1 drops Vetiver		10 drops Amber

Making a room spray

A room spray is useful when you want to include an aroma in your room but not have a constant aroma. Diffuser sticks, potpourri and aroma beads provide a constant aroma while the products are fresh, but a room spray is more controllable and can be used when you want to introduce a smell or mask a nasty odour.

Room sprays contain water as part of their dilution ingredient. To enable perfume oils to disperse in water, you need to include a dispersant. The dispersant suggested in the recipe is polysorbate 20. This is similar to polysorbate 80 used in making scented bath oil (see pages 132–3), but it is lighter, allowing it to form a fine spray. Polysorbate 20 is derived from coconut oil and sorbitol, and has the function of dispersing perfume oils into water without leaving oily droplets.

How to make a scented room spray

This recipe makes approximately 65ml of scented room spray. If you find the aroma of the scented room spray is too strong using 60g water, add more water to dilute it further. The shelf life of your room spray is 12 weeks. You will need the following equipment:

- Scales
- A jug or other container in which to mix the ingredients
- A spoon for stirring
- A bottle with spray attachment

Ingredients
- 2g polysorbate 20
- 60g tepid boiled water or distilled/deionised water
- 2g perfume blend oil (approximately 60 drops)

1. Put the polysorbate 20 into the mixing jug and add a little of the water – about 3–4 tablespoons (approximately 50g). Mix well; it may be a little thick initially.

2. Add your perfume blend oil and continue to mix thoroughly.

3. Gradually add rest of the water until the liquids are thoroughly blended and dispersed.

4. Pour the scented room spray into a suitable spray bottle and add a label so that you can identify the contents of the bottle.

Using your scented room spray
Shake the bottle each time you use it in case the contents have separated. Spray the scented room spray into the air. Avoid spraying it over the surfaces of furniture in case it leaves a mark when it settles.

Room spray recipes
Each recipe below makes 60 drops of perfume oil – approximately 2g – and can be used as the perfume oil in your scented room spray.

Shift	Revive	Fresh Daisy
30 drops Lime	20 drops Bergamot	19 drops Grapefruit
10 drops Eucalyptus	10 drops Orange	3 drops Bay
15 drops Green Apple	5 drops Coriander	20 drops Rose
5 drops Benzoin	5 drops Basil	12 drops Fig
	10 drops Oakmoss	5 drops White Tea
	10 drops Patchouli	1 drop Vetiver
Dizziac	**Warm Embrace**	**Hush**
5 drops Bergamot	8 drops Orange	10 drops Lime
10 drops Neroli	5 drops Mandarin	10 drops Cucumber
20 drops Jasmine	15 drops Rose	5 drops Coriander
20 drops Rose	14 drops Rose Geranium	10 drops May Chang
5 drops Patchouli	8 drops Clove	5 drops Oakmoss
	10 drops Rosewood	20 drops Amber

Making a linen spray

The room spray recipe can also be used for a linen spray. Since you'll be spraying the scented liquid directly onto material rather than into the air, you may want to dilute it further. Using up to 140g water (double the amount used in the room-spray recipe) will still give you perfumed linen.

Using your scented linen spray

Before spraying the perfumed linen spray onto your best fabrics, test it on a piece of material first to ensure it doesn't leave a mark. Your perfumed linen spray contains oils and, depending on the perfume blend you designed, may contain dark-coloured oils. While these won't necessarily leave a mark once the spray has dried, it's best to do a test just to make sure.

Linen spray recipes

Each recipe below makes 60 drops perfume oil – approximately 2g – and can be used as the perfume oil in your heavily diluted linen spray.

Lavender	Pristine	Luxuriate
45 drops Lavender	10 drops Peppermint	24 drops Jasmine
15 drops Rose Geranium	50 drops Cucumber	24 drops Rose
		12 drops Vanilla
Refresh	Sparkle	Awaken
30 drops Lemon	10 drops Bergamot	20 drops Grapefruit
10 drops Bay	10 drops Green Apple	5 drops Watermelon
10 drops Lemon Grass	30 drops Bamboo	10 drops Basil
10 drops Benzoin	10 drops Amber	20 drops Fig
		5 drops Grass

CHAPTER 11

Perfume Blend Formulations

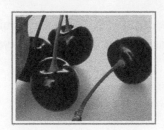

SELECTION OF FAVOURITE BLENDS

Here I have included a selection of my favourite blends. Some are simple, some are more complex; some are more suitable as a light, refreshing daytime spray whereas others are appropriate as a sensual and very special evening perfume. Just to make sure we don't leave anyone out, I have included blends that my husband would wear – although he tells me that I wear more than enough for him to have to worry!

Feel free to modify them as you wish. If you don't have all the oils specified, then try substituting the missing oil for another in the same fragrance family. For example, you might swap amber for benzoin, vanilla for tonka bean or lemon for lime.

Alternatively, swap the oil for a completely different aroma to change the structure of the perfume dramatically. For example, swap amber for rosewood (both base notes, but amber is sweet oriental whereas rosewood is from the woody family), or swap amber for cucumber (cucumber is middle note from the green family) or even amber for bergamot (bergamot is a top note from the fruity citrus family).

There are no hard-and-fast rules here. Just have fun experimenting!

Light daytime blends

Light daytime blends are easy to wear. The following recipes are based on making 2g of the perfume blend (60 drops).Combine any blend formulation with 98g dilutant for a 100g bottle of body spray. Combine any blend formulation with 38g dilutant for a 40g bottle of eau de toilette.

Unique U

This one is a particular favourite of mine. It is a very feminine, floral aroma that is suitable for daytime – especially sunny days, when we eventually get them!

- 20 drops Neroli
- 20 drops Jasmine
- 10 drops Tuberose
- 7 drops Musk
- 3 drops Sandalwood

PF17

A very refreshing, light, fruity daytime spray which is certainly worth the effort you need to put in opening all those bottles.

- 2 drops Lemon
- 3 drops Neroli
- 3 drops Bergamot
- 2 drops Orange
- 2 drops Lime
- 3 drops Apple
- 2 drops Cardamom
- 3 drops Coriander
- 2 drops Geranium
- 3 drops Lavender
- 2 drops Nutmeg
- 4 drops Rose
- 2 drops Rosemary
- 2 drops Tobacco Leaf
- 2 drops Violet
- 2 drops Musk
- 2 drops Labdanum
- 2 drops Benzoin
- 2 drops Cedar
- 2 drops Rosewood
- 2 drops Patchouli
- 2 drops Sandalwood
- 2 drops Vanilla
- 2 drops Vetiver
- 3 drops Amber
- 2 drops Oakmoss

Rohanna

If you aren't keen on floral or sweet fruits, this perfume is delicately scented with flowers without an overall blast of sweet, cloying floral.

- 10 drops Cardamom
- 12 drops Black Tea
- 19 drops Jasmine
- 9 drops White Lily
- 10 drops Sandalwood

Vanille et Fleurs

Translated as 'Vanilla and Flowers', this perfume also has a dash of anise to cut through the floral layer, giving it an interesting twist.

- 8 drops Anise
- 4 drops Frangipani
- 10 drops Rose
- 10 drops Gardenia
- 2 drops Clove
- 10 drops Ylang-ylang
- 14 drops Vanilla

Siri Usiko

A light, refreshing introduction quickly gives way to a sweet, oriental dry-down... this perfume changes as you wear it.

- 20 drops Bergamot
- 20 drops Lilac
- 6 drops Vanilla
- 10 drops Amber
- 4 drops Musk

Shout!

Very refreshing and invigorating. The aroma will uplift and energise.

- 10 drops Orange
- 10 drops Peppermint
- 10 drops Lime
- 20 drops Geranium
- 10 drops Patchouli

Exotic evening blends

The following blends are slightly heavier and more soporific than the daytime blends, but they can be worn as daytime sprays for those who like a bold perfume. Combine any perfume blend formulation with 38g dilutant for a 40g bottle of eau de toilette. Combine any perfume blend formulation with 18g dilutant for a 20g bottle of eau de parfum.

Imposter

This fragrance is neither sweet nor sharp, floral nor fruity. Its careful blend of flowers and fruit are mingled with sweet orientals to create an intriguing, engaging aroma.

- 5 drops Anise
- 15 drops Neroli
- 5 drops Clove
- 6 drops Violet
- 12 drops Hyacinth
- 5 drops Jasmine
- 12 drops Tonka Bean

Cassis et Satis

After the soft introduction of orange blossom, this perfume layers you with silky blackcurrant combined with rose and underpinned with sensual patchouli. It is a wonderful mix of flowers, fruit and woods, leaving a delightful aromatic trail.

- 15 drops Neroli
- 8 drops Blackcurrant
- 32 drops Rose
- 5 drops Patchouli

Diversion

A simple blend that dives straight in with middle to base notes. There is no fruity top layer to awaken your senses; this perfume just explodes with rose, captivating your senses and trapping them in a heady bouquet.

- 20 drops Rose
- 30 drops Amber
- 10 drops Rosewood

Nectaramour

Definitely one for the frivolous perfume-wearer: a charming blend of sweet, fruity delights. It's perfect for a balmy evening as it emerges from the warmth of a summer's day to the sultry heat of a summer night. (Don't be tempted to add more chocolate unless you want to smell like pudding!)

- 8 drops Pink Pepper
- 12 drops Peach
- 6 drops Cherry
- 14 drops Rose
- 10 drops Honey
- 4 drops Patchouli
- 2 drops Amber
- 2 drops Benzoin
- 2 drops Chocolate

Chennai Nights

The very feminine florals entwined with the slightly sour vetiver make this a remarkably easy-to-wear perfume. Leave it to settle and allow the vetiver to succumb to the heady essence of the florals before bottling.

- 26 drops Rose
- 16 drops Jasmine
- 14 drops Ylang-ylang
- 4 drops Vetiver

Viungo Spice

A mysterious perfume where sweet meets spice, it seems to change as you wear it.

- 15 drops Neroli
- 5 drops Strawberry
- 2 drops Cinnamon
- 4 drops Clove
- 14 drops Frankincense
- 10 drops Tonka bean
- 10 drops Vanilla

Blends for men

Having canvassed a selection of men to find out which individual scents they would like in an aftershave, I was pleasantly surprised to find that several were happy to include flowers. When formulating for men, please don't discard any aromas you think are more appropriate for women. Consider using them, but adjust the levels so that they are background aromas. Combine any perfume blend formulation below with 38g dilutant for a 40g bottle of aftershave.

Loco

When suggesting to my husband that nutmeg would make a useful ingredient in a men's aftershave, he muttered something that was difficult to hear completely, but I did make out the words 'mad', 'no' and 'there's no way I would wear that'.

I initially developed this aftershave without the nutmeg, but it wasn't one I was particularly keen on myself. However, adding the nutmeg made a huge difference. The aromatic nuttiness combined with the soft, fruity mandarin set the whole aroma off beautifully. I let him wear it a few times before I told him it contained nutmeg. He still wears it today.

- 15 drops Mandarin
- 15 drops Lavender
- 5 drops Clove
- 15 drops Nutmeg
- 10 drops Amber

Daring

When first sniffing the bottle of leather you may possibly decide not to include it. By all means make this aftershave without the leather, but I urge you to be daring and try it. Instead of adding the scent of saddle or of a new pair of boots, it adds a certain smokiness to the aftershave, instantly transforming it from runner-up category to winner!

- 14 drops Juniper Berry
- 8 drops May Chang
- 14 drops Tobacco Leaf
- 10 drops Vanilla
- 1 drops Chocolate
- 3 drops Leather
- 2 drops Patchouli
- 8 drops Tonka Bean

Hurricane

A good, honest manly aftershave. No prettiness, nothing hidden, no twists or frilly edges – just 100 per cent man.

- 8 drops Anise
- 1 drop Cinnamon
- 12 drops Black Pepper
- 20 drops Basil
- 16 drops Patchouli
- 3 drops Tonka Bean

Red Life

Floral tuberose and neroli are seen off by the woodiness of cedar and sandalwood. Vetiver adds a final dark-forest flourish, making you completely forget that flowers were included at all.

- 10 drops Neroli
- 10 drops Tuberose
- 10 drops Cedar
- 15 drops Sandalwood
- 5 drops Vetiver

24/7

While the coffee fragrance oil is strong and apparent, it absolutely makes this aftershave. I built the perfume around apple, but when I'd added the coffee, I knew I could stop. This grows on you!

- 20 drops Green Apple
- 20 drops Juniper Berry
- 8 drops Coffee
- 12 drops Tonka Bean

5th Day

Fresh and green with a hint of sweetness.

- 11 drops Galbanum
- 9 drops Grapefruit
- 10 drops Coconut
- 10 drops Tobacco Leaf
- 9 drops Cedar
- 11 drops Honey

Manifico

This aftershave works in layers: from the initial fresh burst of citrus, swiftly followed by an interlude of florals, which very quickly succumbs to the aroma of an autumn walk. This combination makes an aroma tempting for male and female.

- 4 drops Bergamot
- 4 drops Grapefruit
- 4 drops Peppermint
- 2 drops Cinnamon
- 10 drops Rose
- 4 drops Leather
- 8 drops Patchouli
- 10 drops Amber
- 4 drops Myrrh
- 10 drops Rosewood

Funza Pumzi

I'm always a little hesitant to reach for ginger as it can add a slightly sour element to a blend. I believe we've harnessed it here because the sweet jasmine offsets it well.

- 15 drops Mandarin
- 10 drops Lemon
- 5 drops Ginger
- 15 drops Lavender
- 15 drops Jasmine

Adige

An all-time favourite that reminds me of a gentlemen's club. It conjures up leather armchairs, broadsheets, decanters, bowler hats and comfortable, happy hearts.

- 17 drops Lime
- 7 drops Mandarin
- 4 drops Ginger
- 12 drops Petitgrain
- 9 drops Lemon Grass
- 4 drops Cardamom
- 3 drops Oakmoss
- 4 drops Vetiver

Unisex blends

I still find it hard to declare that any individual smell is more suitable for a particular gender. Why should rose be more appropriate for a woman and sandalwood for a man? My belief is that it comes down to the wearer's personal preference.

I'd really like to list all perfume blends in the unisex category, but I've resisted and instead, have singled out my favourites that will hopefully be appealing to all, regardless of gender. Combine any perfume blend formulation with 38g dilutant for a 40g bottle of eau de toilette or aftershave.

Riche
Definitely an overall fruity aroma, bordering on green and fresh, with undertones of thatched roof!

- 20 drops Neroli
- 15 drops Lemon Grass
- 20 drops Fig
- 5 drops Vetiver

Dark Sunset
Another of my favourites and one my husband is keen to borrow from me. He says it's his and that *I* should ask to borrow it – but I beg to differ!

- 17 drops Mandarin
- 4 drops Black pepper
- 8 drops Gardenia
- 17 drops Sandalwood
- 14 drops Vanilla

Censure
An easy-to-wear, fresh cologne-type aroma that also makes an excellent room spray.

- 10 drops Orange
- 5 drops Lime
- 5 drops Eucalyptus
- 10 drops Bay
- 5 drops Rose
- 8 parts Violet
- 12 drops Patchouli
- 5 drops Amber

Zing Star Gazer

Sometimes the simple ones are the most memorable. Don't be put off by the volume of peppermint here; the sharp, minty element evaporates, leaving a refreshing new aroma of green fruit.

- 25 drops Orange
- 10 drops Peppermint
- 25 drops Geranium

Tightrope

Live dangerously! In this blend I've taken citrus, herbs, oceanic, green and floral and balanced them into a fresh, lively aroma.

- 8 drops Orange
- 9 drops Geranium
- 15 drops Lavender
- 4 drops Basil
- 8 drops Salty Sea Dog
- 14 drops Tuberose
- 2 drops Oakmoss

Embrace

Let this wonderful aroma give you a friendly hug and pat on the back. Uplifting yet grounding, energising yet calming, this perfume works with your senses. Try it and see for yourself.

- 6 drops Orange
- 14 drops Bergamot
- 3 drops Geranium
- 9 drops Lavender
- 12 drops Rose
- 10 drops Amber
- 6 drops Patchouli

Resources

Training courses, kits, ingredients and packaging
Plush Folly
www.plushfolly.com
Tel: 07851 429 957

Fragrance oils, perfume ingredients and packaging
Sensory Perfection
www.sensoryperfection.co.uk
Tel: 01273 911245 (but prefers email contact: sensoryperfection@gmail.com)

Gracefruit
www.gracefruit.com
Tel: 01324 841353

The Soap Kitchen
www.thesoapkitchen.co.uk
Tel: 01805 622 944

Essential oils
Fresh Skin
www.freshskin.co.uk
Tel: 07846 174 876

ID Aromatics
www.idaromatics.co.uk
Tel: 0113 242 4983

Specialist herbs, gums and resins
G Baldwin & Co
www.baldwins.co.uk
Tel: 020 7703 5550

Organic Herb Trading
www.organicherbtrading.com
Tel: 01823 401 205

Bottles and packaging
Dormex
www.dormex.co.uk
Tel: 01928 703 160

Coloured bottles
www.colouredbottles.co.uk
Tel: 01634 862 839

Index

Also by Sally Hornsey

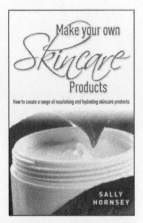

Make Your Own Skincare Products
How to create a range of nourishing and hydrating skincare

If treated and nourished properly your skin will be healthy and glowing, making you feel good and look great.

This book will guide you through creating your own personal range of skincare applications, tailored to your particular skin type – or any body else's. The products made use natural ingredients where possible, and throughout the book you will find details of the purpose and benefits of the ingredients used. You will also learn about ingredients that can be substituted so that you can adapt the recipes to suit your or others' needs.

In this book you will discover how to:

• Choose essential oils that are useful for treating different skin conditions.
• Design and create a range of products including a cleanser, toner, face mask and moisturising cream.
• Identify the ingredients that are beneficial in hand-made skincare products.
• Make informed choices on which ingredients are most appropriate for different skin conditions.
• Make tinctures and infusions to use in your products.
• Store your products to ensure that they are fresh and safe to use.

Sally Hornsey runs **Plush Folly**, a private cosmetic training company, specialising in a range of cosmetic-making workshops, kits and home study courses. Sally has taught many students how to design a range of skincare products for their own use and has given students the skills and knowledge they need to establish a flourishing business.

ISBN 978-1-905862-68-9